EMERGENCY RESPONSE
Workbook

CHECK · CALL · CARE

Second Edition

Mirella G. Pardee, MSN, MA, RN

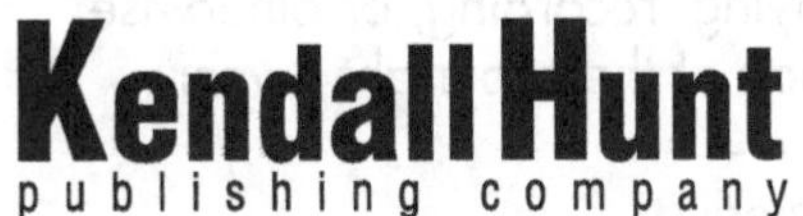

Kendall Hunt
publishing company
www.kendallhunt.com
Send all inquiries to:
4050 Westmark Drive
Dubuque, IA 52004-1840

ISBN 978-1-4652-0490-5

Printed in the United States of America
10 9 8 7 6 5 4 3 2

Contents

Preface

This workbook is designed to supplement the American Red Cross textbook, *Emergency Medical Response* (2011). The content in this workbook meets the 2010 Consensus on Science for CPR and Emergency Cardiovascular Care (ECC) Guidelines. The focus of the workbook revolves around three emergency action steps, ***Check-Call-Care***.

This workbook is structured to align more closely with the content taught in a college level course in first aid. A student who completes this course will have the basic training to assist a person who is ill or injured or who has a life-threatening condition. The activities in the workbook provide a structured format to assist a student who plans to further his or her education as an EMT or paramedic.

Highlights of the workbook include:

- **Learning Activities.** Every chapter includes learning activities that were designed to help students comprehend and retain the most important information from each chapter. Real-life emergency scenarios are included among the variety of learning activities, in order to afford students the opportunity to apply the knowledge and skills that were learned.
- **Expanded Course Content.** Some chapters contain a more thorough discussion of key topics and diagrams to help the student understand important concepts.
- **Skill Check Sheets.** Appendix B contains skill check sheets that were developed to evaluate whether a student is able to meet minimum competencies in the provision of basic emergency care.
- **Algorithms.** Appendix C contains algorithms (decision-making trees) which emphasize the emergency action steps of CHECK-CALL-CARE, for selected skills.

About the Author

Mirella G. Pardee, MSN, MA, RN

Mirella Pardee received her RN diploma from the St. Vincent Hospital School of Nursing, Toledo, Ohio. She graduated from the University of Toledo with a bachelor's degree in nursing and from Wayne State University with a master's degree in nursing. She has been a faculty member at the University of Toledo since 1978, teaching pediatric and medical-surgical nursing classes in the Associate Degree Nursing Program. For the past 12 years, she has taught health education classes, including First Aid, in the Judith Herb College of Education, Health Science and Human Service. She has worked per diem in an area hospital and also as an OB-GYN nurse practitioner for a group of obstetrician-gynecologists. Ms. Pardee is certified as an Emergency Response Instructor Trainer for the Greater Toledo Chapter of the American Red Cross.

Unit 1

Preparatory

1 The Emergency Medical Responder

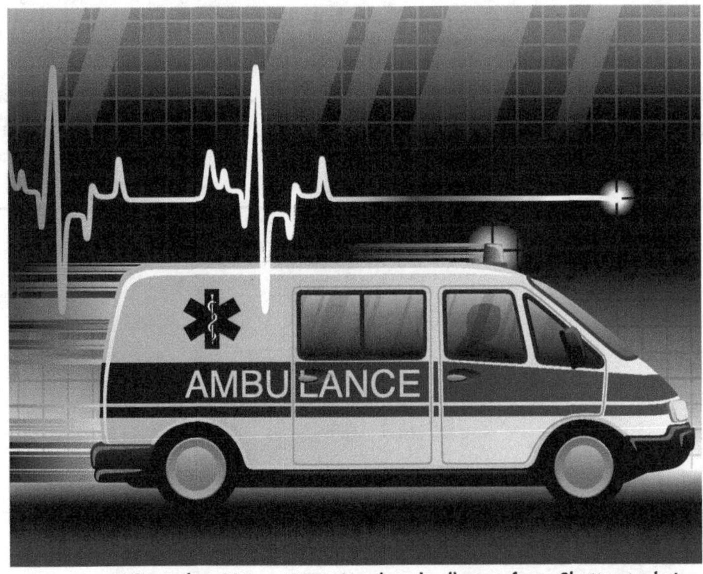

Chapter Significance

The *Emergency Medical Services (EMS)* system is often taken for granted. Dialing three numbers, 9-1-1, immediately connects the caller to an emergency medical dispatcher who must decide which emergency service resource(s) is (are) required, and then send the appropriate resource(s) to the scene of an emergency. Prior to 1973, there was no organized system to handle a variety of emergencies; a person had to contact individual agencies to provide needed services (fire, ambulance, police). Research has shown that ill and injured patients have a much better chance of survival if appropriate emergency care is received prior to hospital transport. Thus, an organized network of community resources and personnel, which became known as the Emergency Medical Services System or EMS, was established to bring medical care quickly to the patient rather than bringing the patient to medical care.

(Continued)

CHECK · CALL · CARE

At the completion of this course, you will be certified as an *Emergency Medical Responder (EMR)*, formerly known as a *First Responder*. Since EMRs are often the first to arrive at the scene of an illness or injury, they are trained to recognize life-threatening conditions and to render appropriate care until more advanced medical personnel arrive.

In this chapter, the student is introduced to the history of the EMS system; the professional levels of EMS certification or licensure; and the role, primary and secondary responsibilities, personal characteristics, and professional behaviors of emergency medical responders. Think back to a time when you or a family member or friend activated the emergency medical services system or made an unexpected trip to the emergency room. Did caregivers treat the ill or injured person with respect and compassion? Did caregivers allay fears exhibited by the ill or injured person, family members, or friends? Did caregivers listen attentively to what the ill or injured person was saying? Were they empathetic to the patient's needs and complaints? Did the caregivers explain what they were doing; were questions adequately answered? The care provided by an emergency medical responder, or other health care professional, can make a lasting impression on an ill or injured patient.

Name: ______________________ Date: ______________

Learning Activities

I. Multiple Choice

1. Emergency medical responders must exhibit certain personal characteristics and professional behaviors that help them in providing care to ill or injured patients. Which of the following statements reflects a personal characteristic?
   a. Keeping fit through daily exercise and a healthy diet
   b. Being able to respond quickly and safely to the scene of an emergency
   c. Being able to provide critical emergency care
   d. Making sure that the scene is safe for oneself and for bystanders

2. Bringing medical care rapidly to the patient rather than bringing the patient to medical care is the basic belief of the
   a. Triage system
   b. Emergency medical services (EMS) system
   c. Emergency medical responder system
   d. National Highway Traffic Safety Administration (NHTSA)

3. The first action of a bystander is to recognize that an emergency exists. Which of the following is the second and most critical action?
   a. Providing care to an ill or injured person
   b. Keeping the scene safe by directing traffic
   c. Activating the EMS system by calling 9-1-1
   d. Transporting the patient to the nearest hospital

4. Who, in the following group of workers, may be an emergency medical responder?
   a. Lifeguards
   b. Camp leaders
   c. Athletic trainers
   d. All of the above

5. Which of the following individuals provides the transition between care given by bystanders and that provided by more advanced medical personnel?
   a. Medical director
   b. Emergency medical responder
   c. Emergency medical technician
   d. Paramedic

6. One of the primary responsibilities of an emergency medical responder arriving at the scene of an emergency is to
   a. Determine whether life-threatening conditions exist
   b. Control and direct bystanders
   c. Transport the patient to the hospital as quickly as possible
   d. Document the patient's condition and the treatment that was given

7. Which of the following statements best describes the emergency medical services (EMS) system?
   a. The EMS system provides an ambulance for patient transport.
   b. The EMS system consists of a network of community resources and personnel organized to provide care for a patient of sudden illness or injury.
   c. The EMS system provides equipment and personnel for removing patients from dangerous locations.
   d. The primary role of the EMS system is to prevent the occurrence of injuries and sudden illness.

II. Short Answer

1. Define the term *emergency medical responder (EMR)*.

2. What is the *EMS system*?

3. Give examples of individuals who can serve as emergency medical responders.

4. List the six primary responsibilities of an EMR.
   1.
   2.
   3.
   4.
   5.
   6.

5. Upon arriving at the scene of an emergency, what is your first responsibility as an emergency medical responder?

6. List the five secondary responsibilities of an EMR.
   1.
   2.
   3.
   4.
   5.

7. What is meant by the term *medical direction* (also known as *medical oversight*)?

8. Who is responsible for providing medical direction (also known as *medical oversight*)?

9. What is a *standing order*?

10. Define the term *scope of practice*.

11. Identify the four professional levels of EMS certification or licensure.

    a. Which type of EMS provider has the most in-depth level of training?

12. EMR certification lasts for ________________years.

13. Standing orders are known as ________________________medical control.

III. Crossword Puzzle

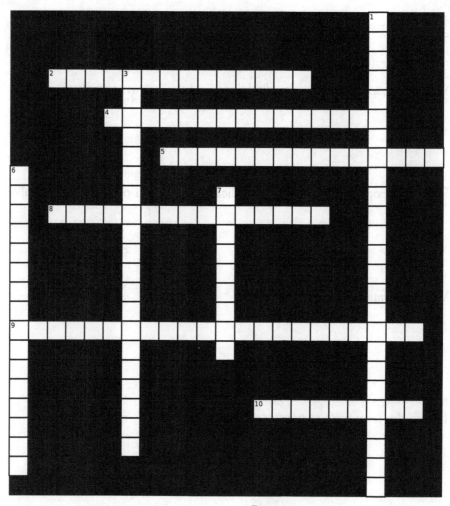

Across

2 Issued by the medical director allowing specific skills to be performed or specific medications to be given in certain situations.

4 Emergency medical care provided before a patient arrives at a hospital or medical facility.

5 A physician who assumes responsibility for the care of injured or ill persons provided in out-of-hospital settings.

8 The range of duties and skills that the EMR is allowed and expected to perform.

9 A type of medical direction in which care can be provided without speaking to a physician.

10 Standardized procedures to be followed when providing care to injured or ill patients.

Down

1 A person trained in emergency care, often the first trained professional to respond to emergencies.

3 The physician speaks directly with emergency care providers at the scene of an emergency.

6 The monitoring of care provided by out-of-hospital providers to ill or injured persons, usually by a medical director.

7 A person with more in-depth training than AEMT.

2 The Well-Being of the Emergency Medical Responder

Expanded Chapter Content

- The Immune System and the Chain of Infection
- Alternate Method for Removing Gloves

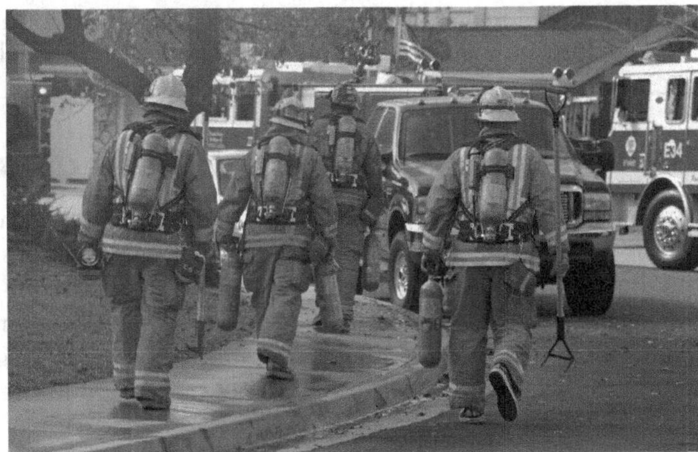

Chapter Significance

Rendering care to an ill or injured patient can expose an emergency medical responder to potentially infectious bodily fluids. Although a variety of pathogens exist that can cause disease, *bloodborne pathogens* present the greatest risk to emergency care providers. The bloodborne pathogens of primary concern are *hepatitis* B (HBV), *hepatitis* C (HCV), and *human immunodeficiency virus* (HIV). The focus of the first part of this chapter is describing the immune system and its functions; describing the four conditions which must be present for the spread of disease; the four ways in which pathogens enter the body; methods to reduce the spread of disease including *body substance isolation* (BSI), *personal protective equipment* (PPE), *engineering controls*, and *work practice controls*. The role and responsibilities of the *Occupational Safety and Health Administration* (OSHA), a federal agency whose function is to promote the safety and health of American workers who may come into contact with blood or other bodily fluids as a result of their job, is discussed.

CHECK • CALL • CARE

The second part of this chapter deals with the emotional aspects of providing care, specifically stress incurred by emergency medical responders as they deal with serious illness, injury, and death in the daily execution of their duties. In order for an EMR to carry out the duties of the job, he or she must be physically and mentally fit. Emergency medical responders must recognize warning signs of stress and develop healthy coping mechanisms to prevent "job burnout." Failure to do so may cause an EMR to experience an emotional crisis, called a *critical incident stress*, in which the ability to be objective and render appropriate care is hampered.

A critical incident stress can also occur among health care workers in a hospital. The Toledo Hospital/Toledo Children's Hospital has a Critical Incident Stress Management (CISM) Team 24 hours per day to assist employees with abnormally stressful work situations. Several incidents have been identified as being particularly stressful to employees: severe injury of a child or multiple patients, suicide, dealing with difficult or hysterical family members, and multiple traumatic events within a short period of time. More than 25 trained employees from a variety of backgrounds make up the CISM team: nursing, patient representatives, social workers, and chaplains. These trained individuals provide on-scene support, *defusion*, and formal *debriefings* for employees.

The Immune System and the Chain of Infection

The immune system is responsible for keeping you safe from disease. White blood cells and antibodies are the body's defenses that destroy disease-causing pathogens. Although a pathogen may enter the body, that doesn't necessarily mean that the person will get sick. In order for disease to develop, all links in the ***Chain of Infection*** must be present and in sequential order. The Chain of Infection contains the four elements necessary for disease transmission (infectious agent, means of transmission, portal of entry, susceptible host), along with two links not mentioned in the textbook: reservoir and portal of exit.

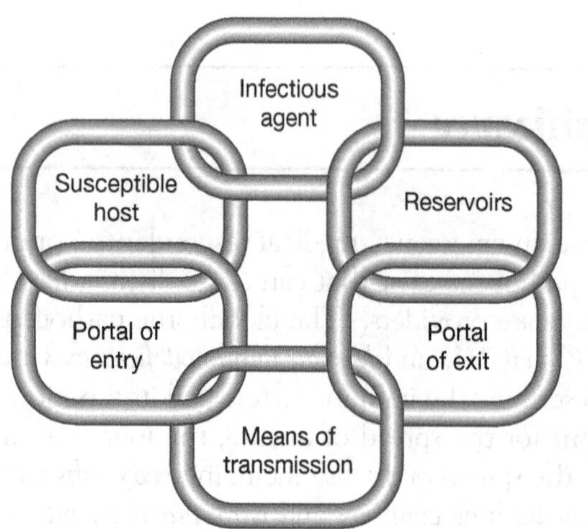

Infectious Agent: Pathogen (bacteria and viruses).

Reservoir: Place where pathogens live (human beings, soil, air).

Portal of Exit: Ways by which pathogens leave a person's body.

Means of Transmission: How pathogens are transmitted from person-to-person or animal-to-person.

Portal of Entry: Ways by which pathogens enter a person's body.

Susceptible Host: Person vulnerable to disease.

Chain of Infection

The first link, ***infectious agent,*** refers to the classification of disease-causing agents, such as protozoa, fungi, bacteria, viruses, rickettsia, prions, yeasts, and parasitic worms.

The second link, ***reservoir,*** is the usual place in which the infectious agent lives and multiplies. Reservoirs may be human, animal, or environmental. Human reservoirs are two types: individuals who are infected with the infectious agent and are sick; and ***carriers***, individuals who have the infectious agent in their body but are not sick. Carriers can present more risks for disease transmission because these individuals do not appear sick, and therefore, their activities are not restricted. Animal reservoirs have the same descriptions as human reservoirs. Environmental reservoirs can include plants, soil, air, and water.

Portal of exit, the third link, is the route by which the infectious agent may escape from the human or animal reservoir. The most common portals of exit are through the respiratory, genitourinary, digestive, and integumentary (skin) systems, and also through the placenta. The respiratory portal of exit is the most important and the one most difficult to control. Many diseases, such as the common cold, influenza, tuberculosis, measles, and mumps are spread through this portal. The genitourinary portal of exit pertains to sexually transmitted diseases including syphilis, gonorrhea, chlamydia, and HIV/AIDS. The digestive system portal of exit can include secretions from the mouth or anus causing a variety of diseases such as salmonella, hepatitis A, and shigella. The skin forms a protective barrier against infection. When the skin is broken through bites, cuts, or needle punctures, infectious agents can exit and cause diseases such as chickenpox, smallpox, malaria, hepatitis B, hepatitis C, and HIV. A pregnant woman can transmit an infectious agent through the placenta to her fetus, such as HIV and cytomegalovirus (CMV).

The fourth link, ***means of transmission,*** bridges the gap between portal of exit and portal of entry. A disease-causing agent must enter the body through the correct portal of entry in order for an individual to become infected. The two basic modes of transmission are ***direct transmission*** and ***indirect transmission***. Direct transmission occurs immediately. Droplet spread is considered direct transmission and many respiratory diseases are spread this way. Indirect transmission can occur through animate or inanimate mechanisms. An animate mechanism involves a vector (mosquitoes, ticks, fleas, and rabid animals), while inanimate mechanisms involve a vehicle such as food, water, or objects contaminated with blood or bodily fluids.

The fifth link, ***portal of entry,*** is usually the same as the portal of exit from the reservoir. It is possible, however, for an infectious agent to escape one person's respiratory tract yet cause a skin infection in another person. If the person with the skin infection handles food, the infectious agent can get into the food and cause "food poisoning" in people who eat the prepared food.

The last link, ***susceptible host***, refers to the health of the individual's immune system through genetic factors or specific acquired immunity. Our genetic makeup can protect us from some diseases. For example, you may know of individuals who are always sick or "catch" an illness very easily while others rarely get sick. Individuals can experience immunity to disease in several ways. The first is called ***innate (natural) immunity***, which refers to one's genetic predisposition, natural barriers such as the skin, and cells within the immune system. When an infectious agent (*antigen*) enters your body and you get sick with the disease (for example, chickenpox), your body makes *antibodies* against that antigen to protect you against getting the same disease twice. This is called ***acquired immunity***. There are two types of acquired immunity: acquired active and acquired passive. ***Acquired active immunity (adaptive immunity)*** can result from receiving a vaccination (immunization) or from having a disease. Having the disease or receiving a vaccine triggers the body to produce antibodies against that infectious agent. If at a later time you come in contact with that infectious agent, you won't get sick. ***Passive acquired immunity (passive immunity)*** is passed from the mother to her fetus and lasts for only a short period of time.

To stop the spread of disease, one or more of the six links in the chain of infection must be broken. Links can be broken through BSI, following standard precautions, and using PPE when providing care.

The most dangerous pathogens for those who provide care to ill or injured patients are those present and transmitted through contact with human blood. These are called *bloodborne* pathogens and include, but are not limited to, hepatitis B virus (HBV), hepatitis C virus (HCV), and human immunodeficiency virus (HIV).

Body substance isolation (BSI) refers to self-protection against all body fluids and substances. As an emergency medical responder, you must assume that all bodily fluids are a possible source of infection and take necessary precautions to avoid coming into contact with them. EMS personnel routinely follow BSI precautions, even if blood or bodily fluids are not immediately visible. In order to decrease the risk of infection, ***personal protective equipment* (PPE)** is used. PPE refers to equipment and supplies that prevent the emergency medical responder from coming into contact with potentially infectious material and can include gloves, mask, protective eyewear, and a waterproof, disposable gown. The PPE that you choose depends on the nature of the care that will be rendered. ***Standard precautions*** are safety measures which are taken to prevent exposure to blood or bodily fluids. Standard precautions combine BSI and universal precautions and assume that any bodily fluid may be infectious.

Check-Call-Care Skill: Alternate Method for Glove Removal

Step 1

- Grasp the wrist area of the glove on one hand and lift up to break the seal.

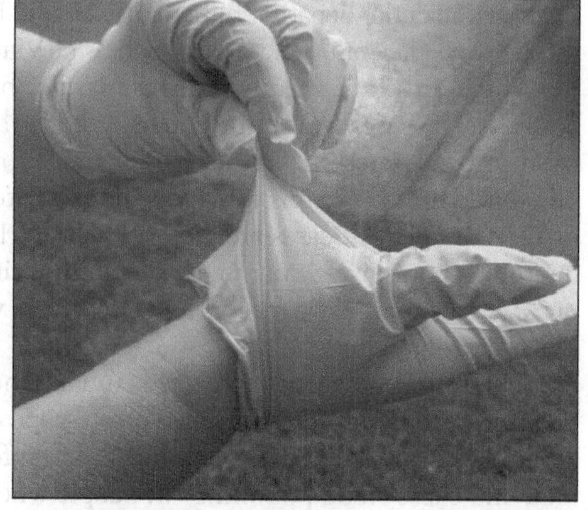

Step 2

- Pull the first glove partially off the hand just to the fingers.

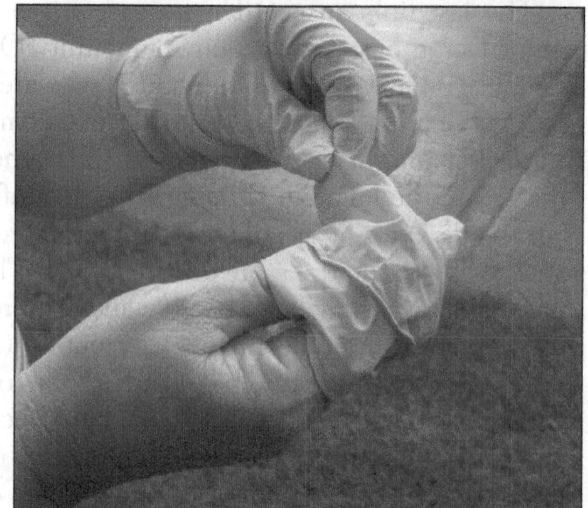

Step 3

- With your partially gloved hand, grasp the wrist area of the other glove and pull it slowly off the hand so that the glove is inside out.

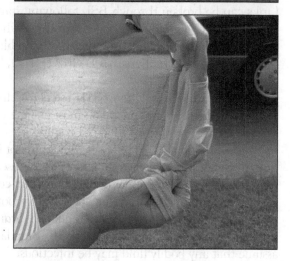

Step 4

- Holding the inside out glove, place it on top of the partially removed first glove, being careful not to touch the outside of the glove with your bare hands.

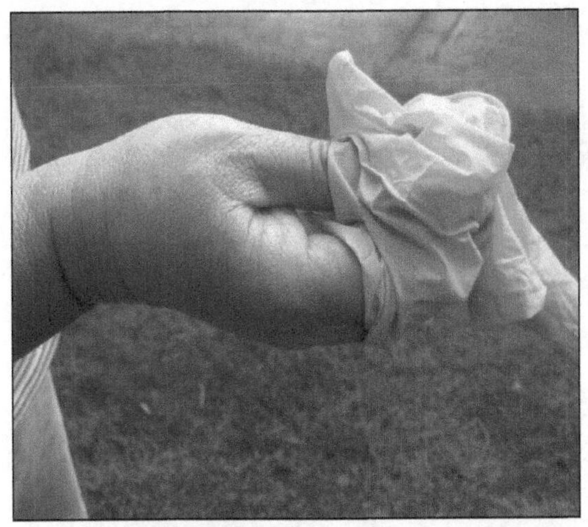

Step 5

- Touching only the inside surface of both gloves, pull them off your hand.
- Dispose of the gloves in an appropriate container.
- Immediately wash your hands with soap and water.

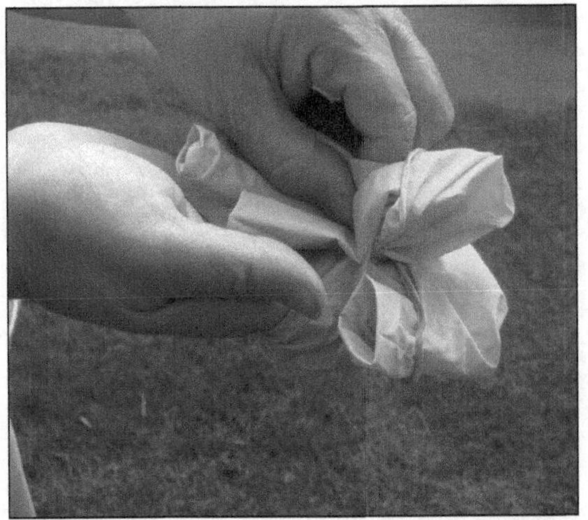

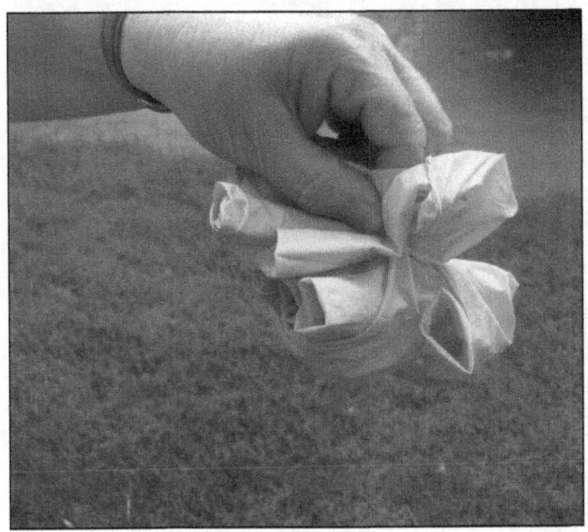

Name: ______________________________ Date: ____________

Learning Activities

I. Multiple Choice

1. A type of pathogen that depends on another living organism to live and reproduce is a
   a. Bacterium
   b. Protozoan
   c. Virus
   d. Fungus

2. The transmission of disease from a patient to an emergency medical responder requires four conditions. Which of the following is one of those conditions?
   a. The pathogen must be present in the patient's body.
   b. The portal of entry must be correct.
   c. The EMR must be susceptible to the pathogen.
   d. All of the above are conditions.

3. The component of the immune system that protects a person against infection is the
   a. Red blood cell
   b. White blood cell
   c. Platelet
   d. Serum

4. Through which of the following routes can the hepatitis B virus be transmitted?
   a. Direct contact
   b. Indirect contact
   c. Droplet transmission
   d. Both a and b

5. You are providing care to a patient at the scene of a motor vehicle collision. The patient has a cut on his arm that is bleeding; the blood is flowing in a steady stream. Which of the following personal protective equipment should you wear to prevent disease transmission?
   a. Protective eyewear
   b. Disposable mask
   c. Disposable gloves
   d. Disposable gown

6. An effective solution for cleaning up a blood spill is _______ of liquid chlorine bleach to 1 gallon of water.
   a. 1 pint
   b. 1 cup
   c. 1 ½ cups
   d. ¼ cup

7. If you are exposed to bodily fluids while providing care, your first action is to
   a. Try and find out if the patient has a disease present
   b. Notify your supervisor or any involved medical personnel
   c. Be tested at a hospital
   d. Wash the contaminated area thoroughly with soap and water

8. A pathogen may enter the body in which of the following ways?
   a. Direct contact
   b. Indirect contact
   c. Droplet
   d. All of the above

9. Jaundice is a disease of the
   a. Liver
   b. Heart
   c. Brain
   d. Spleen

10. When providing care, which of the following actions would protect the emergency medical responder against bloodborne pathogens?
    a. Using disposable supplies such as bandages and dressings instead of gloves
    b. Using personal protective equipment during care
    c. Washing hands only before providing care
    d. Checking the patient's medical record to determine whether the patient has an infectious disease

11. Which stage of the grieving process involves a promise of something in exchange for a reversal of the previous condition?
    a. Anger
    b. Bargaining
    c. Denial/disbelief
    d. Acceptance

12. Which of the following assumes that all body fluids, secretions, and excretions are potentially infective?
    a. Universal precautions
    b. Body substance isolation precautions
    c. Personal protective equipment
    d. Standard precautions

13. While providing care to a patient, some of the patient's body fluids splash into your eyes. What is the first action to take?
    a. Flush your eyes with clear water for 20 minutes.
    b. Wash your face with soap and water.
    c. Apply an antibiotic ointment to the eyes.
    d. Rinse the eyes with a disinfectant solution.

II. Short Answer

1. What is a pathogen? Give several examples of pathogens.

2. Define the term *antibody*.

3. Define the term *immunization/vaccination*.

4. What conditions, as identified in the chain of infection, are necessary for an infectious disease to be transmitted?

5. What are the four ways by which diseases are transmitted?
   1.
   2.
   3.
   4.

6. How is *malaria* transmitted?

7. Provide the mode of transmission for each of the following diseases:

Disease	Mode of transmission
AIDS	
TB	
Meningitis	
Hepatitis B	
Hepatitis C	

8. What does the acronym *OSHA* stand for? Why is it important?

9. Define the term *body substance isolation (BSI)*.

10. What does the term *PPE* stand for?

11. Provide examples of precautions and practices which can be used to protect oneself from exposure to any type of bodily substance.

12. When giving ventilations to a patient who isn't breathing, which personal protective equipment is most important to use to protect you and the patient from disease transmission?

13. Explain the term *engineering control* and give three examples.

14. What is the first step to take in removing gloves?

15. Individuals who provide emergency care can experience high levels of stress.
    A. What is meant by *critical incident stress*?

    B. List five signs of critical incident stress.

16. An informal session held immediately after an emergency incident that allows an emergency medical responder to vent anger or frustration is called a critical incident stress ________.

17. As a general rule, an emergency medical responder should always attempt to resuscitate a patient who has no pulse and is not breathing. Under what situations should resuscitation not be attempted?

18. What are the five stages of grieving?
    1.
    2.
    3.
    4.
    5.

III. True or False

_______ 1. All infectious diseases are communicable.

_______ 2. You do not need to wash your hands after wearing medical gloves to provide care to a patient.

_______ 3. Rabies and Lyme disease are examples of vectorborne illnesses.

_______ 4. An emergency medical responder can develop tuberculosis by coming in contact with an infected patient's blood.

_______ 5. Even with a healthy immune system, an emergency medical responder may develop an infectious disease.

_______ 6. Touching an object that has been contaminated by the blood of an infected patient is called direct contact transmission.

_______ 7. Equipment and supplies that protect emergency medical responders against becoming infected are called personal protective equipment (PPE).

_______ 8. Safeguards that isolate or remove hazards from the workplace are called engineering controls.

IV. Scenarios

Scenario 1

You are driving home on the interstate after spending the holiday with family. It is late evening and the earlier rain has begun to freeze, making the street slippery. Suddenly, the minivan in front of you begins to swerve and slide, rotating 360 degrees. It crosses the median where it is struck and pushed back into the roadway and into a ravine. You immediately pull off onto the shoulder of the road. (Questions 1–4 refer to scenario 1.)

1. What are the possible dangers to you in this scenario?

2. What are the possible dangers to the patient(s) in this scenario?

3. Assuming that the scene is safe, what is the first action that you would take?

4. When you call 9-1-1, what information should you provide to the dispatcher?

Scenario 2

You are summoned to respond to a call for injuries from a fall. You arrive to find a small child lying motionless on the ground. He had fallen out of a third story window. Two women are standing by the child. One woman, the child's mother, is kneeling next to the child crying and screaming. It appears as though the child is dead. As you try and get close to the child, the mother refuses to let you near the child, screaming at you to stay away. (Questions 1 and 2 refer to Scenario 2.)

1. Can you treat the child without the mother's consent? Provide a rationale for your answer.

2. How can you help the mother deal with the death of her child while awaiting the arrival of EMS?

V. Web-Based Exercise (Extra Credit Assignment)

Go to the following website: http://www.ehs.okstate.edu/modules/index.htm. Click on ***bloodborne pathogens*** and view the presentation in an online, PowerPoint or Word document format. After you have reviewed the information, go to www.ehs.okstate.edu/modules/bbp/bbpquiz.htm to take the 10 question quiz; print the results and give to your instructor. You only need to type in your first and last name on the top of the quiz.

3 Medical, Legal, and Ethical Issues

Expanded Chapter Content

- Negligence
- Good Samaritan Laws

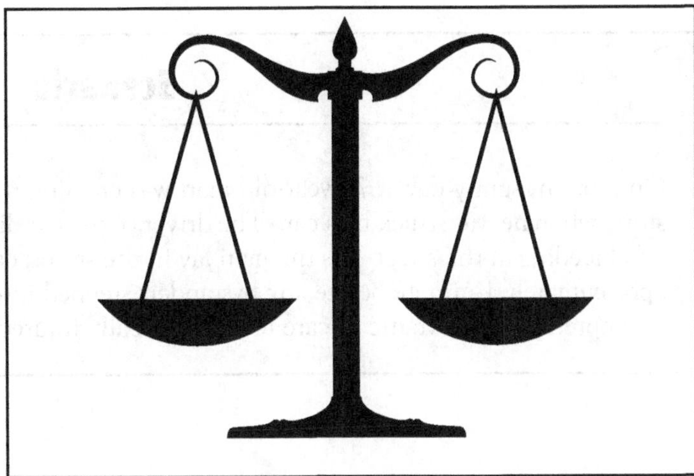

Chapter Significance

As an emergency medical responder, you will be in a position to help someone who suddenly falls ill or becomes injured. You will want to help the person and not cause any further harm. However, what if the care you provide does not have a positive outcome? Could you have exposed yourself to possible legal action?

When you step into your professional role as an emergency medical responder, you will be faced with many difficult questions on a regular basis.

- Should you stop at the scene of a car accident and treat any patients when you are not on duty?
- Should you provide information to the news reporter who approaches you, praising your heroic efforts in saving a person's life?

Continued

- Should you treat a child who appears injured when the parents or legal guardian are not available?
- How can you determine whether providing care to a patient would be futile?
- What should you do if you determine a person needs your help but refuses it?

This chapter provides the emergency medical responder with general medical, legal and ethical principles that can be used to guide care when these questions arise.

Scenario

On a bright sunny day, a 70-year-old man was crossing the street, after a brief trip to the grocery store, when he was struck by a car. The driver of the car did not stop, leaving the man unconscious and bleeding in the street. As the man lay in the street, cars passed him without stopping. It took approximately 1 minute before any bystanders stepped into the street to get a closer look. No one attempted to divert traffic or care for the critically injured man.

While this scenario is disturbing to most people, we need to try to understand why bystanders who witnessed the accident did not attempt to help this critically injured, elderly man.

Many reasons can be offered but, in today's litigious society, many people are reluctant to help out in emergency situations. People fail to act for a variety of reasons: concern regarding doing something wrong; not knowing what to do; fear of disease transmission; not wanting to get involved in other people's problems; and fear of being sued. If a lawsuit is filed against an emergency medical responder (the Defendant), the charge made by the Plaintiff (the patient or family of the patient) will usually be one of ***negligence.***

I. Negligence: What Is Negligence?

Negligence is "the failure to follow a reasonable standard of care, thereby causing injury or contributing to injury or damage to another" (American Red Cross, 2011, p. 53).

You can find comfort in knowing that very few emergency medical responders have been sued and the burden of proof rests on the shoulders of the Plaintiff. The Plaintiff has to prove four elements in order for a lawsuit charging negligence to be successful. These four elements are: duty, breach of duty, cause, and damage.

The element of duty not only includes the ***duty to act*** but also the duty to act appropriately, following the accepted *standards of care* and acting as another reasonable emergency medical responder would in a similar situation.

As to the first aspect of duty, the question centers around whether the emergency medical responder owed a legal duty of care to the plaintiff or patient. Emergency medical responders, which include police officers and firefighters, perform emergency care as part of their job descriptions; they owe a duty to the public, especially to the population whom they serve. They have a legal obligation to respond and provide care at the scene of an emergency while they are "on the job." However, one needs to separate a moral versus a legal duty to act. An individual "on duty" has a legal obligation to act, whether in a volunteer or paid position. Once the job/shift has ended, the duty to act has also ended; an emergency medical responder should morally respond to an emergency but there is no legal obligation to do so.

As to the second part of the duty to act, the question centers around whether the emergency medical responder acted appropriately, according to the *standards of care* established by both national and state authorities and the laws which govern the *scope of practice* for the EMR.

The second element of negligence is ***breach of duty***. Did the emergency medical responder fail to fulfill (breach) the duty? Did the emergency medical responder fail to act (act of omission) or fail to act appropriately (act of commission) in a specific situation?

The third and fourth elements of negligence, ***cause*** and ***damage***, are best described together. Did the actions or lack of actions by the EMR cause physical or emotional injuries to the patient? Providing evidence which links the causation and the damages is the most difficult issue to prove in a court of law. The question that will be asked is, "Had it not been for the actions of the emergency medical responder, would the patient have suffered the injury or died?"

II. Good Samaritan Laws

Return once again to the scenario at the beginning of this chapter. A man was critically injured, yet none of the bystanders offered assistance or even called 9-1-1. They may have chosen not to become involved because of a fear of legal action if they did something wrong and caused further harm to this patient.

In order to encourage people to stop and render care to patients at the scene of an emergency, every state has enacted laws or regulations which protect health care professionals and other rescuers from being sued when they are providing emergency "out of hospital" care. In some states, the law has also been expanded to cover the general public.

In legal terms, a Good Samaritan refers to someone who voluntarily renders care in an emergency to an injured person without expecting anything in return. Generally, if the Good Samaritan makes an error while giving emergency care, he or she cannot be held legally liable for damages in a court of law. However, protection or immunity from legal liability under the Good Samaritan law must satisfy certain conditions: (1) Care is given at the scene of an emergency; (2) care is rendered willingly or voluntarily; (3) care is not reckless or careless (negligent); (4) the "volunteer" acts in good faith without an expectation of being paid a fee or reward for the care provided; and (5) the patient does not, when able, object to being helped.

Good Samaritan laws vary from state to state. Therefore, it is important to become familiar with the laws of the state in which you practice and understand the degree of protection that is provided.

Name: ______________________ Date: __________

Learning Activities

I. Multiple Choice

1. The range of duties and skills an emergency medical responder is expected to provide to a patient in a given situation is called
   a. Duty to act
   b. Scope of practice
   c. Standard of care
   d. Code of ethics

2. The failure to act as a similarly trained emergency medical responder would in a similar situation is called
   a. Breach of duty
   b. Duty to act
   c. Causation
   d. Damage

3. Protecting a patient's privacy by sharing information about the patient with only those who need to know, in order to continue treatment of a patient, is referred to as
   a. Invasion of privacy
   b. Confidentiality
   c. Disclosure
   d. Accountability

4. Showing compassion and carrying out your responsibilities as an emergency medical responder in a professional manner are examples of a(n)
   a. Duty to act
   b. Scope of practice
   c. Legal liability
   d. Ethical responsibility

5. Unless an illness or injury to a child is life threatening, the emergency medical responder must first obtain consent from a parent or guardian. This type of consent is known as
   a. Presumptive consent
   b. Expressed consent
   c. Implied consent
   d. Minor's consent

6. Good Samaritan laws protect a person from legal liability when providing care in an emergency under which of the following conditions?
   a. The person obtains verbal consent from the patient.
   b. The person identifies himself or herself by name to the patient and states his or her level of training.
   c. The person offers help with the expectation of being reimbursed for services.
   d. The person acts in good faith within his or her scope of practice.

7. You arrive at the scene of a robbery at a convenience store where the employee was stabbed in the chest. Law enforcement personnel have secured the scene. Which of the following statements is appropriate in providing care to the patient in this situation?
   a. Assume control of the situation as soon as you arrive.
   b. To protect yourself from bloodborne pathogens, have law enforcement personnel clean up blood around the patient.
   c. Take care not to disturb any item at the scene.
   d. Obtain immediate access to the patient upon your arrival.

8. Prior to providing care to a patient, what is the first thing that you should do as an emergency medical responder?
   a. Ask the patient how the injury occurred.
   b. Identify yourself to the patient by name and level of training.
   c. Describe the injuries that you see to the patient.
   d. Explain in detail the care you intend to provide to the patient.

9. You are providing care to a male patient who has fallen off the roof of a shed. The patient is conscious. Which of the following actions should you take first?
   a. Obtain consent from the patient to provide care.
   b. Ask the patient about any complaints of pain.
   c. Check the patient's pulse and breathing rates.
   d. Ask the patient what happened when he fell.

10. An emergency medical responder determines that a patient is competent under which of the following circumstances?
   a. The patient is capable of identifying an appropriate health care proxy.
   b. The patient understands that any information that is shared will remain private.
   c. The patient gives verbal or nonverbal acceptance of the treatment to be given.
   d. The patient understands the emergency medical responder's questions and the implications of decisions.

11. As an emergency medical responder, you are expected to provide care based on specific criteria which is called the
   a. Standard of care
   b. Duty to act
   c. Scope of practice
   d. Good faith action

II. Short Answer

1. Identify the four elements that must be proven by a patient for any negligence lawsuit to be successful.

   1.

   2.

   3.

   4.

2. Describe the similarities and differences between two advance directives: the living will and the durable power of attorney for health care.

3. Describe how you would obtain consent from a competent, adult patient.

4. The legal document which describes how a person wants to be cared for in the event of a medical emergency is a/an ________________________________.

5. Touching and providing care to a competent patient who has refused the offer of emergency assistance may lead to a charge of ________________________.

6. The legal document which gives another person the authority to consent and make health care decisions for someone who is unable to do so is a/an ______________________________.

III. Matching

Column A

_____ 1. Acronym for legal document which gives another person the authority to consent to health care for a person who is not able to make health care decisions on his or her own.

_____ 2. Acronym used to designate the withholding of life-sustaining procedures.

_____ 3. Permission to treat given by the patient verbally or in writing.

_____ 4. Sharing medical information about the patient only with law enforcement personnel and health care providers at the emergency scene.

_____ 5. The legal term meaning "responsibility."

_____ 6. Threat or attempt to inflict harm on another person.

_____ 7. Deviation from the accepted standard of care, contributing to injury or damage to the patient.

_____ 8. Ending care of a patient without ensuring that care will continue at the same level or higher.

_____ 9. The range of duties and skills an emergency medical responder is allowed to legally perform which are established by state laws and regulations.

_____ 10. Ability to understand information provided and the consequences of decisions made.

_____ 11. The "yardstick" against which the actions of the emergency medical responder will be measured.

_____ 12. Type of consent applied to unresponsive or unconscious patients.

_____ 13. Failing to act or acting inappropriately, outside of the emergency medical responder's scope of practice.

_____ 14. Legal obligation to provide emergency medical care.

_____ 15. Provides emergency care in good faith.

Column B

A. Abandonment
B. Battery
C. Breach of duty
D. Confidentiality
E. Competence
F. Duty to act
G. DNR
H. DPOA
I. Expressed consent
J. Implied consent
K. Liability
L. Negligence
M. Scope of practice
N. Standard of care
O. Assault
P. Good Samaritan

IV. Scenario

On your way home from work, as a volunteer firefighter, you witness the car in front of you suddenly swerve and crash into the roadside ditch. You stop and see the driver slumped over the steering wheel. (Questions 1–4 refer to the scenario).

1. Do you have a duty to act? Provide rationale for your answer.

2. If you make a decision to stop and render care, your first priority should be to
   a. Assess the scene for hazards
   b. Assess the patient's level of consciousness
   c. Control any bleeding from open wounds
   d. Look for any life-threatening conditions

3. What possible dangers might be present at the scene of this motor vehicle accident?

4. After an ambulance has arrived and the patient has received care, a reporter from a local television station stops you to ask some questions. How would you respond to the reporter's request?

V. Web-Based Exercise (Extra Credit Assignment)

Good Samaritan laws differ from state to state. Go to the website www.cprinstructor.com/legal.htm. Then click on "EMS, CPR, AED Legal Database-case law." From the list of states, select one state and answer the following questions about the Good Samaritan law for that state.

Which state are you reporting on?

1. Define these terms as they are used in the context of the law.

   - Immunity

   - Civil liability

   - Reasonably prudent person

2. Who is protected by the law in the selected state?

4 The Human Body

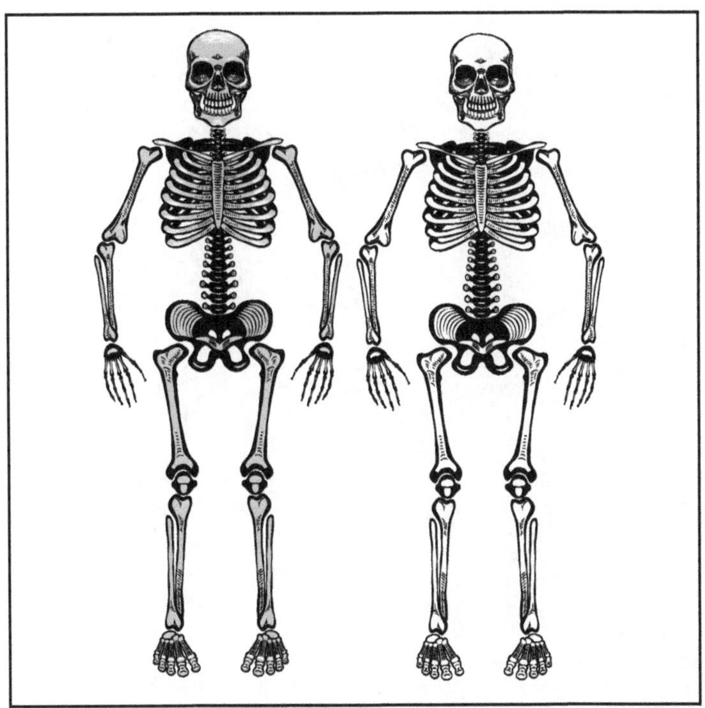

Chapter Significance

As an emergency medical responder, you must have a basic understanding of the structure and function of human body systems in order to perform an accurate assessment of ill or injured patients. How can you identify whether a person has a life-threatening condition, such as a heart attack, if you are not familiar with the anatomy and physiology of the circulatory (cardiovascular) system?

Having an understanding of how each body system normally works will help you identify problems that develop when a body system is not working properly. Understanding the body's structures and how they work is not only essential to accurate assessment, but also to the provision of proper emergency care.

CHECK ▪ CALL ▪ CARE

In addition to providing information on the basic anatomy and physiology of various body systems, this chapter also introduces emergency medical responders to common *combining forms*, *prefixes*, and *suffixes* that make up medical terms so that an EMR can accurately document findings and relay pertinent information to more advanced medical personnel. Anatomical terms, body cavities, and terms related to patient positioning are also discussed.

Name: ______________________________ Date: ____________

Learning Activities

I. Multiple Choice

1. A small structure which keeps food and liquids out of the lower respiratory tract during swallowing is the
   a. Epiglottis
   b. Larynx
   c. Tonsil
   d. Uvula

2. The function of white blood cells is to
   a. Stop bleeding
   b. Transport oxygen
   c. Prevent infection
   d. Secrete hormones

3. The structure where gas exchange between atmospheric air and blood takes place is the
   a. Alveolus
   b. Bronchus
   c. Larynx
   d. Trachea

4. The normal resting breathing rate for an adult is
   a. Less than 12 breaths per minute
   b. 12–20 breaths per minute
   c. 20–30 breaths per minute
   d. 30–40 breaths per minute

5. The brachial artery is located in the
   a. Leg
   b. Lower arm
   c. Upper arm
   d. Neck

6. A person who has diabetes has a problem with the ____________________ system.
   a. Digestive
   b. Endocrine
   c. Nervous
   d. Musculoskeletal

7. A pulse is correctly located over a(an)
   a. Arteriole
   b. Capillary
   c. Vein
   d. Artery

8. A patient who was shot was found lying on his back. The medical term for this position is
   a. Abdominal
   b. Lateral
   c. Prone
   d. Supine

9. The thoracic cavity contains which of the following structures?
   a. Brain and spinal cord
   b. Spleen and intestines
   c. Heart and lungs
   d. Stomach and liver

10. _______________ are structures found at joints that connect one bone to another.
   a. Articulations
   b. Ligaments
   c. Muscles
   d. Tendons

11. Blood vessels that carry oxygen-poor blood from the body back to the heart are called
   a. Arteries
   b. Arterioles
   c. Capillaries
   d. Veins

12. The body's **first** line of defense against infection is part of the __________ system.
   a. Circulatory
   b. Respiratory
   c. Musculoskeletal
   d. Integumentary

13. Which body system helps to regulate body temperature through heat production?
   a. Genitourinary
   b. Digestive
   c. Respiratory
   d. Musculoskeletal

14. Which body system transports oxygen and nutrients to cells of the body and removes waste products?
   a. Digestive
   b. Circulatory
   c. Endocrine
   d. Respiratory

15. The body systems that work together to supply adequate levels of oxygen to tissues of the body are
   a. Circulatory and respiratory
   b. Digestive and respiratory
   c. Integumentary and circulatory
   d. Nervous and circulatory

16. Which of the following terms refers to a body part that is closest to the trunk of the body?
    a. Distal
    b. Medial
    c. Lateral
    d. Proximal

17. The plane which divides the body horizontally is called the _____________ plane.
    a. Axial
    b. Coronal
    c. Sagittal
    d. Frontal

18. Which of the following body systems is responsible for fighting disease?
    a. Respiratory system
    b. Endocrine system
    c. Integumentary system
    d. Immune system

19. _______________ are structures that attach muscle to bone.
    a. Joints
    b. Tendons
    c. Ligaments
    d. Fascia

II. Short Answer

1. A patient who is lying face-down is in a __________________ position.

2. If a body part is above another body part, its location is ____________________.

3. The combining form which means "heart" is ______________________.

4. The term *medial* refers to the __________________ of the body while the term *lateral* refers to the __________________ of the body.

5. The term that describes a structure which is located towards the head is __________________ or ______________________; the term that describes a structure which is located towards the feet is ____________________ or ______________________.

6. The prefix which means "fast" is ________________.

7. The prefix that means "excessive or above normal" is ________________________.

8. List the five body cavities.
    1.
    2.
    3.
    4.
    5.

9. List the three vital organs: _____________, _____________, _____________.

10. The larynx is commonly known as the ____________________.

11. Name the two main anatomical systems of the nervous system.

    1.____________________________________

    2.____________________________________

12. The structure that separates the thoracic cavity from the abdominal cavity is the ________________________.

13. The arteries which supply oxygenated blood to the heart muscle are the ______________ arteries.

14. The largest part of the integumentary system is the _______________.

15. Blood vessels which carry oxygenated blood from the heart to the body are ____________________.

16. The largest organ of the body is the ________________________________.

17. Another name for the collarbone is the ________________________________.

5 Lifting and Moving Patients

Expanded Chapter Content/ARC Updates

- Patient Positioning:
  - Modified H.A.IN.E.S recovery position

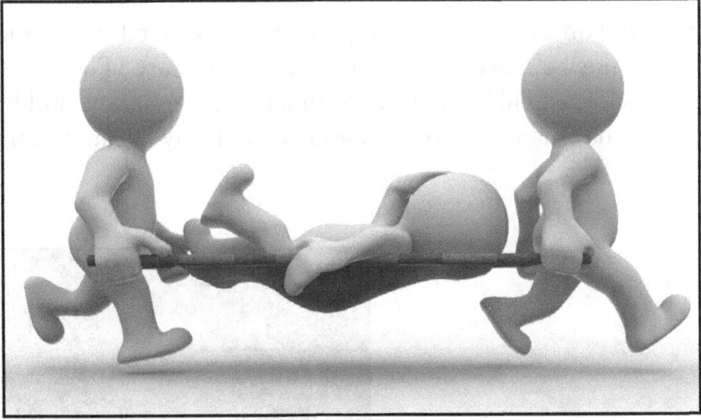

Chapter Significance

The general rule of thumb when you are the first medically trained person to arrive at an emergency scene is to treat patients where they are found. Do not move patients unless it is absolutely necessary, especially if you suspect from the patient's position or the nature of the injury, that the patient may have a spinal injury. Unnecessarily moving a patient can cause further injury to the patient and can also cause harm to the emergency medical responder.

In some emergency situations, however, the patient must be moved immediately, prior to assessment and treatment. These situations include: (1) the presence of scene hazards which pose an immediate danger to you and the patient; (2) the need to gain access to patients who require lifesaving care, when multiple patients are ill or injured; and, (3) the patient's position or location prevents the delivery of appropriate care.

This chapter describes different ways to lift and move patients safely, using proper *body mechanics*. No single method is the best way to move all patients. One needs to take into account many factors when making a decision to move a patient, including the type of injuries the patient has. The safest and easiest method will be the one which moves the patient rapidly without causing injury to the emergency medical responder or the patient.

Expanded Chapter Content

A. Patient Positioning

In most situations, emergency medical responders will assess and care for patients in the position in which they are found. However, it may be necessary for the emergency medical responder to change a patient's position in order to facilitate patient assessment or to make the patient more comfortable.

Turning from a *prone* (face down) position to a *supine* (face up) position: If the patient is unresponsive and found face down, he or she must be turned face up so that a thorough assessment can be done and a transfer can be made to a backboard.

B. Modified H.A.IN.E.S. (High Arm IN Endangered Spine) Recovery Position

If an unconscious, breathing patient is suspected of having a head, neck, or back injury, the patient should not be moved unless absolutely necessary. Placing a patient into a modified H.A.IN.E.S recovery position should only be performed if you are alone and have to leave the patient to call for help or if you cannot maintain an open and clear airway because of fluids or vomit (Figure A).

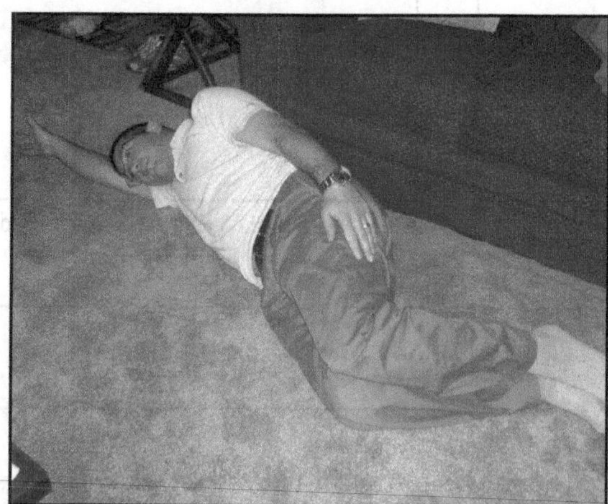

Figure A
Modified H.A.IN.E.S. recovery position

Sources

American Heart Association and the American National Red Cross (2010). Part 17: First aid: 2010 American Heart Association and American Red Cross Guidelines for First Aid. *Circulation* 122:S934-S946. http://circ.ahajournals.org/content/122/18_suppl_3/S394

Name: ______________________________ Date: ______________

Learning Activities

I. Multiple Choice

1. Of the following situations, which one is least likely to involve moving the patient before care can be provided?
   a. A patient involved in a motor vehicle collision lying next to a smoking vehicle
   b. A patient who was painting a house and fell off the ladder onto the grass
   c. A patient who has collapsed inside the doorway of a burning building
   d. A patient slumped over the car's steering wheel who has no breathing or pulse

2. Which of the following statements best reflects the principles of moving a patient?
   a. The power grip allows for maximum hand stability and strength.
   b. You should pull rather than push whenever possible.
   c. Reaching over a distance of 10 inches should be avoided.
   d. The squat lift is preferred over the power lift when moving a patient.

3. The best method to use when moving a patient with a suspected head, neck, or spinal injury is the
   a. Shoulder drag
   b. Ankle drag
   c. Firefighter's drag
   d. Blanket drag

4. Of the following emergency moves, which one can be performed by one rescuer with an unconscious patient?
   a. Direct lift
   b. Firefighter's carry
   c. Shoulder drag
   d. Seat carry

5. In the modified H.A.IN.E.S. recovery position, the patient's head and neck are supported on
   a. A folded blanket
   b. A long backboard
   c. The rescuer's arm
   d. The patient's raised arm

6. What is the minimum number of rescuers needed to safely logroll a patient with a possible head, neck, or spinal injury?
   a. 2
   b. 3
   c. 4
   d. 5

7. In most situations, care should be provided to patients positioned
   a. On their back
   b. On their right side
   c. How they were found
   d. On their left side

8. A patient lives on the third floor of an apartment building and needs to be moved to an ambulance. There is no elevator in the building and the staircase is narrow. Which of the following devices would be most appropriate to use in moving this patient?
   a. Wheeled stretcher
   b. Stair chair
   c. Short backboard
   d. Scoop stretcher

II. Short Answer

1. Describe three situations in which an emergency medical responder must move a patient.

   1.

   2.

   3.

2. What does the acronym *H.A.IN.E.S.* stand for?

3. Under what conditions would the emergency medical responder place a patient in a modified H.A.IN.E.S. recovery position?

4. Under what condition is it acceptable for an emergency medical responder to use restraints on a patient?

III. Matching

Column A

_____ 1. The most basic emergency move used with injured conscious patients.

_____ 2. An emergency move in which the patient's arms are pulled over the rescuer's shoulders and the patient is carried on the rescuer's back.

_____ 3. A one-rescuer emergency move for patients suspected of having spinal injuries.

_____ 4. A method of moving conscious patients by cradling the patient between two rescuers.

_____ 5. An emergency move in which the patient is pulled to a sitting position and lifted across the rescuer's shoulders.

_____ 6. A minimum of three emergency medical responders is needed to complete this move.

Column B

A. Clothes drag
B. Direct ground lift
C. Firefighter's carry
D. Pack-strap carry
E. Two-person seat carry
F. Walking assist

IV. Scenarios

Scenario 1

A 54-year-old woman has jumped from the second floor of her home, trying to escape smoke and fire. She is lying on the ground with a bleeding wound to her forehead and complaining of chest pain. (Questions 1 and 2 refer to Scenario 1.)

1. Name at least five factors you would consider before moving this woman?

2. Which emergency move would be the most appropriate to use with this patient? Provide rationale for your answer.

Scenario 2

As you ride along the bike trail, you are tired but relaxed. You must have ridden at least 10 miles. As you round a sharp curve, you abruptly swerve to avoid a young woman sprawled in the middle of the path. From the looks of things, she appears to have been rollerblading and fell. She is in obvious pain, cradling her bent arm close to her chest. She has a large abrasion over her knee and multiple scrapes and scratches. You stop your bike in order to help. (Questions 1 and 2 refer to Scenario 2.)

1. Would you move the patient before providing care? Provide a rationale for your answer.

2. Would you activate EMS for this patient? Provide a rationale for your answer.

Unit 2

Assessment

6 Scene Size-Up

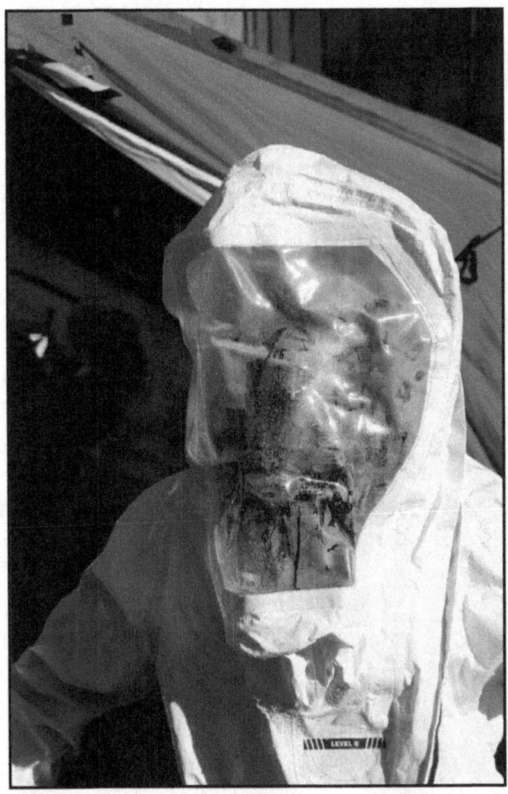

© TFoxFoto, 2011. Used under license from Shutterstock, Inc.

Chapter Significance

Taking the time to evaluate the scene of an emergency can make the difference between the emergency medical responder being able to assist a patient in need or the emergency medical responder becoming a patient himself. Sometimes dangers are not readily apparent, such as toxic fumes from *hazardous materials (HAZMAT)* such as natural gas. The EMR will be alert to dangers in an emergency scene by using the senses of hearing, smelling, feeling, and seeing. The EMR must look for

dangers at the scene of every emergency: unstable structures; downed electrical wires; the potential for explosions or fires in car accidents; and dangers from oncoming vehicles. One of the secondary responsibilities of emergency medical responders is to protect bystanders from dangers such as traffic or fire. By thoroughly evaluating the emergency situation, all needed resources are dispatched to the scene by the *communication center (dispatch)* when EMS is called.

Name: ______________________________ Date: ______________

Learning Activities

I. Multiple Choice

1. The physical event that caused the injury is called
   a. Nature of the injury
   b. Mechanism of injury
   c. Kinematics of trauma
   d. Chocking

2. Which of the following may indicate the presence of hazardous materials?
   a. Clouds of vapor
   b. Unusual odors
   c. Spilled liquids or solids
   d. All of the above

3. Individuals who transport hazardous materials are required by the U.S. Department of Transportation to print placards identifying
   a. The specific hazardous material
   b. The hazardous material name or number
   c. The dangers of the hazardous material
   d. All of the above

4. Which of the following actions should an emergency medical responder do first when arriving at the scene of an emergency?
   a. Complete a primary assessment
   b. Size up the scene
   c. Summon more advanced medical personnel
   d. Obtain the patient's consent to provide care

5. You arrive at the scene of an emergency and are sizing up the scene. Which of the following would be considered least hazardous to you?
   a. A downed electrical wire
   b. The smell of gasoline
   c. Large and small pieces of broken glass
   d. A damaged vehicle on the side of the road

II. Short Answer

1. How far away should you park from a fire?

2. List the four guidelines that an EMR should follow at the scene of an emergency to ensure personal safety and the safety of bystanders.
   1.
   2.
   3.
   4.

3. Clothing and specialized equipment that provides protection to the EMR from substances that can cause illness or injury is called ______________ ______________ ______________.

4. List the four situations which may require an emergency move.
   1.
   2.
   3.
   4.

5. Placing blocks or wedges against the wheels of a vehicle is called ______________.

6. A type of injury in which a person is struck by or falls against a blunt object and the skin is not broken is referred to as a ______________ ______________.

7. Define the term *hematoma*.

8. Define the term *kinematics of trauma*.

9. An EMR notices a patient sitting in a tripod position. What types of problems would the patient most likely be experiencing?

10. List six signs that indicate the presence of hazardous materials.
    1.
    2.
    3.
    4.
    5.
    6

III. True/False

_______ 1. The very first action taken by an emergency medical responder at the scene of an emergency is to ensure that the scene is safe for bystanders and rescuers.

_______ 2. An emergency medical responder should not approach a scene containing hazardous materials unless PPE are available.

_______ 3. A hematoma can result from a blunt trauma injury.

_______ 4. A patient should not be moved unless absolutely necessary.

_______ 5. Ideally, a patient should be moved only after he or she has been assessed and properly cared for.

IV. Scenarios

Scenario 1

A Putnam County man who drove to the scene of a one-vehicle crash to offer assistance was killed by an electric shock when he stepped on a downed power line along a darkened road. The man was home when the power went out briefly. Believing that the power outage was due to an accident, he drove about one-half mile when he saw that an SUV had struck a utility pole, severing the pole and bringing the wires down. The man got out of his vehicle to offer assistance and stepped on the live wire as he was walking toward the SUV. The man was declared dead at the scene. (Questions 1–3 refer to Scenario 1.)

1. What are the factors from this scenario that placed the man's life in danger?

2. What should the man have done prior to leaving his house?

3. When the man arrived at the scene of the crash, what information should he have given to the 9-1-1 dispatcher?

Scenario 2

A 14-year-old boy was killed in Durham, North Carolina, after he climbed an electrical tower near a high school. The boy and his two friends were hiking in the woods near the tower when the boy decided to climb it, despite warning signs detailing high voltage. One of the boy's friend begged him not to climb the tower but he didn't listen. Soon a loud pop was heard by the neighbors. The boy was electrocuted and fell off the tower. The two friends frantically called 9-1-1 and met emergency crews at the opening to the woods. (Questions 1 and 2 refer to Scenario 2.)

1. What scene safety hazards may be present in this situation?

2. If you were the first emergency medical responder to arrive on the scene, what would be the first action to take in this situation?

7 Primary Assessment

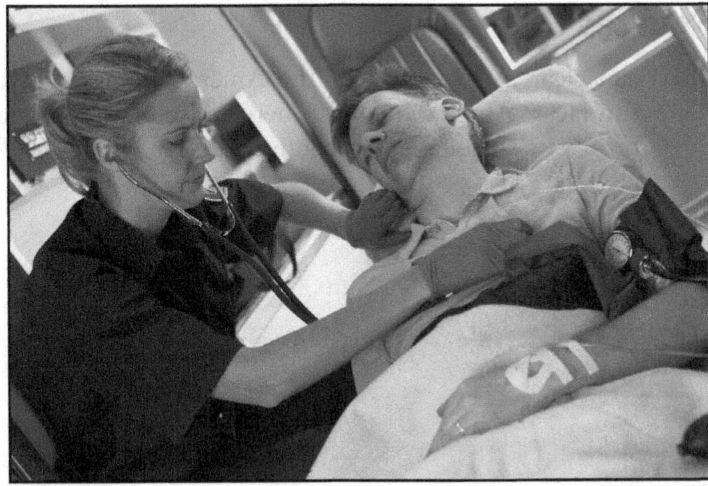

© Monkey Business Images, 2009. Used under license from Shutterstock, Inc.

Expanded Chapter Content

- Witnessed sudden collapse of an adult

Chapter Significance

This critically important chapter provides the foundation upon which the assessment and subsequent care of an ill or injured patient by an emergency medical responder takes place. You will learn how to recognize levels of consciousness, how to open a patient's airway and determine if the patient is breathing and has a pulse. You will be able to look for signs, based on the patient's symptoms that can help alert you to the nature of the illness and the mechanism of injury.

In Chapter 3, you were introduced to the term *standard of care* in the performance of your job duties. In this chapter, you will learn how to follow these standardized guidelines when conducting a *primary (initial) assessment* of a patient so that you are not negligent in carrying out your actions.

CHECK · CALL · CARE

Expanded Chapter Content: Witnessed Sudden Collapse of an Adult

Please note that in a witnessed sudden collapse of an adult, quickly check for the presence of breathing and a pulse. If neither is present, begin chest compressions. The two initial ventilations are eliminated.

Sources

American Heart Association and the American National Red Cross (2010). Part 17: First aid: 2010 American Heart Association and American Red Cross Guidelines for First Aid. *Circulation* 122:S934-S946. http://circ.ahajournals.org/content/122/18_suppl_3/S394

Name: ______________________________ Date: ______________

Learning Activities

I. Multiple Choice

1. Conducting a primary (initial) assessment in every emergency situation is important because
   a. It protects you from liability should a lawsuit arise
   b. It will help you identify conditions that are an immediate threat to the patient's life
   c. It enables you to protect the patient and bystanders from dangers at the scene
   d. All of the above

2. Of the following patients, which one has a life-threatening problem?
   a. An 18-year-old female with a fever who vomited three times in 24 hours
   b. A 45-year-old jogger experiencing severe ankle pain after a morning run
   c. A 58-year-old executive complaining about sharp pain in his side when he takes in a deep breath
   d. A 3-year-old girl found floating unconscious in a swimming pool

3. A normal adult takes between ___and ___breaths per minute.
   a. 6, 12
   b. 12, 20
   c. 20, 24
   d. 24, 28

4. Signs and symptoms of abnormal breathing include
   a. Flaring of the nostrils
   b. Quiet, regular breaths
   c. Whistling or gurgling sounds
   d. Both a and c

5. How often should artificial ventilations be given to an adult who is not breathing but has a pulse?
   a. Once every 15 seconds
   b. Once every 10 seconds
   c. Once every 5 seconds
   d. Once every 3 seconds

6. How often should ventilations be given to a child who is not breathing but has a pulse?
   a. Once every 15 seconds
   b. Once every 10 seconds
   c. Once every 5 seconds
   d. Once every 3 seconds

7. How often should ventilations be given to an infant who is not breathing but has a pulse?
   a. Once every 15 seconds
   b. Once every 10 seconds
   c. Once every 5 seconds
   d. Once every 3 seconds

8. You assess a patient and find that he is able to answer your questions appropriately. Using the AVPU mnemonic, you would give this patient the letter
   a. A
   b. V
   c. P
   d. U

9. After sizing up the scene, you conduct a primary assessment of the patient. Which of the following do you evaluate first?
   a. Airway
   b. Breathing
   c. Circulation
   d. Responsiveness

10. For which of the following situations would you activate EMS?
    a. A patient with an airway obstruction who is coughing forcefully
    b. A patient with a minor cut on the forearm that is bleeding slightly
    c. A patient with an open leg wound with the bone protruding
    d. A patient with intermittent abdominal pain

11. You and another rescuer find an adult lying on the floor. One rescuer leaves to summon EMS. You conduct a primary assessment and find that the patient is unconscious, has a pulse but not breathing. Which of the following actions would be appropriate for you to take?
    a. Give one ventilation every 5 seconds.
    b. Give the patient five back blows followed by five chest thrusts.
    c. Perform a finger sweep of the patient's mouth.
    d. Perform CPR.

II. Short Answer

1. What are the five components of the *primary (initial)* assessment?

2. What is the purpose of the *primary (initial)* assessment?

3. What are the four main components to consider during a *scene size-up*?

   1.

   2.

   3.

   4.

4. State five situations in which EMS should be activated.

   1.

   2.

   3.

   4.

   5.

5. When forming a *general impression* of the patient, what six questions should an EMR ask oneself?

   1.

   2.

   3.

   4.

   5.

   6.

6. Define the terms *sign* and *symptom* and give an example of each.

Sign:	**Example**
Symptom:	**Example**

7. State and define each letter in the mnemonic AVPU.

   A =

   V =

   P =

   U =

8. When opening a patient's airway, the EMR finds that the patient is wearing dentures. What action, if any, should the EMR take?

9. The technique used to open the airway in a patient without a head, neck, or back injury is the ______________________________ technique. The technique used to open the airway in a patient with a suspected head, neck, or back injury is the ____________________.

10. The EMR should look, listen, and feel for breathing and feel for a pulse for no more than ______________.

11. The term which means that the patient is not breathing is ______________ ______________.

12. Define the term *stoma*.

13. Define the term *agonal gasps*.

14. If the emergency medical responder finds a patient with agonal gasps, what care should be given?

15. A patient who has a bluish discoloration to the skin from lack of oxygen is said to be ______________________.

16. A patient with pale, cool, clammy and moist skin as a result of inadequate oxygenation is said to be ________________________.

17. The three signs of an abnormal pulse are
    1.
    2.
    3.

18. Define the term *perfusion*.

19. How is capillary refill assessed? Why is it assessed?

20. Define the term *vital signs (signs of life)*.

21. Where should an emergency medical responder check for a pulse in an unconscious adult, child, and infant?

22. In assessing skin characteristics, what is an emergency medical responder looking for?

III. True or False

_______ 1. A circulation check involves checking for a pulse, checking for severe bleeding, checking for broken bones.

_______ 2. To help the emergency medical responder determine a patient's level of consciousness, the mnemonic AVPU is used.

_______ 3. A patient who is "alert" must also be oriented.

_______ 4. The very first action taken by an emergency medical responder at the scene of an emergency is to ensure that the scene is safe for bystanders and rescuers.

_______ 5. A general impression is formed during the physical exam.

_______ 6. If a patient is unresponsive, an emergency medical responder should look for a medical alert tag.

_______ 7. Using capillary refill to assess adequate blood flow is more reliable in children under the age of 6.

IV. Crossword Puzzle

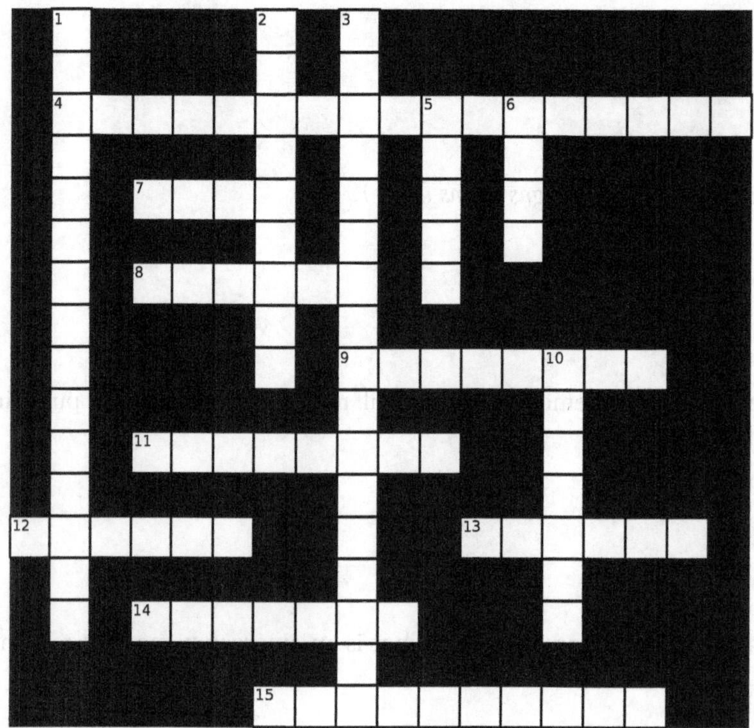

Across

4 The process used to quickly identify those conditions that represent an immediate threat to the patient's life.

7 The mnemonic used to describe levels of consciousness.

8 The name of the artery located on the thumb side of the wrist.

9 The bluish discoloration of the skin due to inadequate oxygenation.

11 The name of the artery located in the upper arm.

12 Before an emergency medical responder can check for breathing, the ___must be opened.

13 The blood vessel in which a pulse is found.

14 The name of the artery located in the neck.

15 Consists of level of consciousness, breathing, and circulation including pulse and skin characteristics.

Down

1 An estimate of the amount of blood flowing through capillary beds, such as those in the fingertips.

2 The circulation of blood through the body or through a particular body part.

3 The technique for opening an airway.

5 An opening in the neck which allows a person to breathe.

6 Something seen, heard, or felt by an emergency medical responder during the primary (initial) assessment.

10 What the patient tells you they are experiencing.

8 History Taking and Secondary Assessment

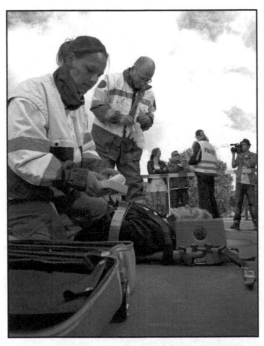

Chapter Significance

This chapter teaches the emergency medical responder how to gather information related to the patient's illness or injury, called the *chief complaint*. Once the chief complaint has been identified, a *physical examination* is performed. The mnemonic *DOTS* remind the emergency medical responder about what to look for while performing the physical examination. Most patients do not need a complete head-to-toe physical examination. Often, emergency medical responders conduct a focal assessment, focusing only on the patient's specific illness or injury. Any life-threatening condition must be treated prior to performing a physical examination.

CHECK · CALL · CARE

The mnemonic *SAMPLE* helps the EMR remember what questions to ask the patient when taking a history. These standardized guidelines protect the emergency medical responder from *negligence* and ensure that the care provided to the patient falls within the *scope of practice* and follows an appropriate *standard of care*.

Name: ______________________________ Date: ______________

Learning Activities

I. Multiple Choice

1. To perform a physical examination on an adult patient, which of the following techniques would be appropriate?
   a. Begin by visually inspecting the entire body, starting with the head.
   b. Gently rub your hands over the patient's arms and legs to feel for possible broken bones.
   c. To make sure that there aren't any injuries to the chest, ask the patient to take a deep breath and exhale, unless he or she complains of chest pain.
   d. All of the above are appropriate.

2. The purpose of performing a physical exam is to
   a. Find injuries that are not immediately life threatening
   b. Determine whether the patient is bleeding severely
   c. Determine whether any hazardous conditions exist
   d. Find out the patient's name and address

3. You are walking with a neighbor along a trail when she trips on a branch and turns her ankle. She seems to have injured the ankle but does not want you to call for help. After a few minutes of sitting on the ground, she wants to stand up. What should you do?
   a. Call EMS because she may have a broken ankle.
   b. Leave her alone on the trail while you get your car to drive her to the hospital.
   c. Help her to stand up so that you can reassess her condition.
   d. Call her doctor for advice.

4. In conducting a *SAMPLE* history, the "P" reminds the emergency medical responder to ask about
   a. Previous hospitalizations
   b. Prior calls to the EMS system
   c. Pain
   d. Past medical history

5. A *focal assessment* should be performed
   a. Only when the injury is limited to a specific body region
   b. When the EMR has a limited time frame in which to conduct a head-to-toe assessment
   c. When the patient refuses a head-to-toe assessment
   d. On a child or infant

6. The "S" in *DOTS* reminds the emergency medical responder to look for
   a. Signs and symptoms
   b. Swelling
   c. Shortness of breath
   d. Seizures

7. In the mnemonic *OPQRST*, which letter refers to what makes the pain better or worse?
   a. P
   b. Q
   c. R
   d. S

8. The primary reason for conducting an *ongoing assessment* is to
   a. Gather more information regarding the injury or illness
   b. Look for any changes in the patient's condition
   c. Give the EMR something to do while awaiting the arrival of the EMS
   d. Reassure the patient and family members

9. You are obtaining a SAMPLE history from a patient with abdominal pain. Which statement made by the patient correlates with the "L" in a SAMPLE history?
   a. "I drank a glass of apple juice about two hours ago."
   b. "I take an antacid occasionally for stomach pain."
   c. "I was treated for a stomach ulcer three years ago."
   d. "The pain has gotten worse over the past five hours."

10. While interviewing a patient, you observe her grimacing and holding her abdomen as she changes her position. Which of the following questions would be least appropriate for an emergency medical responder to make in this situation?
    a. "Does your abdomen feel strange?"
    b. "Why did you make that face just now?"
    c. "Are you feeling uncomfortable?"
    d. "Are you having pain in your belly?"

11. Which of the following is an example of a chief complaint?
    a. "I have a history of high blood pressure."
    b. The patient drank 8 ounces of water 1 hour ago.
    c. The patient fell from a height of 7 feet.
    d. "I was having really severe pain in my chest."

II. Short Answer

1. What does the mnemonic *DOTS* mean?

   D =
   O =
   T =
   S =

2. What does the mnemonic *SAMPLE* stand for?

   S =
   A =
   M =
   P =
   L =
   E =

3. What does the mnemonic *OPQRST* stand for?

O =
P=
Q=
R=
S=
T=

4. List four signs and symptoms of abnormal breathing.
   1.
   2.
   3.
   4.

5. A normal pulse rate for an adult is between ______ and ______ beats per minute.

6. Performing a physical examination involves the techniques of ________________ (looking); ____________________ (feeling); ____________________ (listening).

7. When placing a blood pressure cuff over a patient's arm, the cuff is placed over the ____________________artery.

8. A blood pressure (BP) is expressed as two numbers. The top number is the systolic pressure and the bottom number is the diastolic pressure. What does the diastolic blood pressure reflect?

9. An *ongoing assessment* is performed every __________minutes on unstable patients and every __________minutes on stable patients.

III. True/False

_______ 1. When performing a physical examination on a patient, ask the patient to move painful body parts carefully.

_______ 2. It is necessary to perform a head-to-toe physical examination on every patient.

_______ 3. When conducting a physical examination, the EMR should use the techniques of inspection, palpation, and auscultation.

9 Communication and Documentation

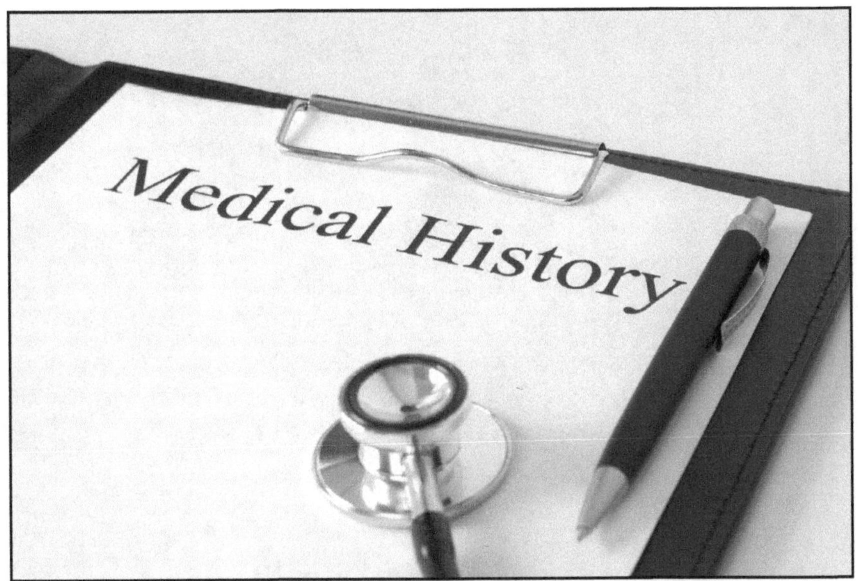

Chapter Significance

Before rendering care to an ill or injured patient, the emergency medical responder will have to elicit information from the patient, family, or bystanders regarding the nature of the emergency. In order to gather information, the EMR must establish rapport with the patient and gain the patient's trust. Effective communication ensures that adequate information is gathered from the patient and that this information is transferred to more advanced medical personnel.

Remember that the information the EMR gathers and writes down in the *prehospital care report* (PCR) is considered confidential and is protected by HIPAA (Health Information Portability and Accountability Act). The document is also considered a legal document of the care that was rendered and could be called into question should a lawsuit arise.

CHECK · CALL · CARE

Name: ______________________________ Date: ______________

Learning Activities

I. Multiple Choice

1. Which statement is the best example of an open-ended question?
   a. "Are you experiencing any pain now?"
   b. "What problems are you experiencing?"
   c. "Is the pain steady or does it come and go?"
   d. "Is a friend or family member here who can stay with you?"

2. Which of the following techniques would be most beneficial for the emergency medical responder to use when interviewing patients?
   a. Speak slowly and clearly.
   b. Use medical terms so the patient understands your level of training.
   c. Address your questions to family members because the patient may not be able to respond to your questions.
   d. Limit questions to yes or no answers so as not to tire the patient.

3. Ways in which the emergency medical responder can adapt the physical environment to facilitate communication include
   a. Get down to the patient's eye level
   b. Establish eye contact with the patient
   c. Address the patient by name
   d. All of the above

4. The segment of the prehospital care record (PCR) that is most frequently falsified is
   a. The physical exam
   b. Treatment
   c. Medication wasted
   d. Time on call

5. Documentation procedures are established by
   a. State regulations or local policy
   b. The National Emergency Medical Responder Register
   c. The National Safety Council
   d. The National American Red Cross unit

II. Short Answer

1. What does HIPAA stand for? Why is HIPAA important related to documentation in the prehospital care report (PCR)?

2. If an emergency medical responder made an error of omission or commission of care, how should the situation be handled?

3. When an emergency medical responder receives verbal medical direction, the order should be repeated back word-for-word. This is called the __________ ______________.

4. ________________ is the point of contact between the public and emergency medical responders.

5. The *prehospital care report (PCR)* is also known as the ____________ or ______________.

III. True/False

_______ 1. One of the best ways to establish a patient's level of consciousness, ability to communicate, and mental status is to ask the patient questions.

_______ 2. A closed question is one in which the patient answers only yes or no.

_______ 3. When interviewing a patient, it is best to avoid asking "why" questions.

_______ 4. Cultural differences may impact the care provided by an emergency medical responder.

_______ 5. The documentation by an emergency medical responder is considered a legal document.

_______ 6. Documentation should include both objective and subjective comments.

IV. Scenario

You arrive at the home of an elderly couple where the husband has fallen during the night. The man is lying on his left side on the floor of the bedroom screaming in pain. His left leg is bent at an odd angle. His wife is at his side, holding her husband's hand, and crying. Questions 1-3 refer to scenario 1.

1. Before you begin to render care to the patient, your first responsibility is to
   a. Make sure the scene is safe
   b. Introduce yourself to the couple
   c. Ask the wife what happened
   d. Splint the patient's leg

2. An example of an open-ended question to ask the patient is:
   a. "Are you having pain now?"
   b. "Did you hit your head when you fell?"
   c. "Did you have any trouble walking before this happened?"
   d. "Can you tell me what happened?"

3. When the emergency medical responder begins interviewing the couple, he discovers that they have a limited command of the English language. Which of the following steps would be most appropriate to take in this situation?
   a. Limit the number of questions asked of the couple.
   b. Ask the couple if they have a friend or family member who can translate for them.
   c. Do nothing since there will be translators available at the hospital.
   d. Notify your direct supervisor of the situation.

Unit 3

Airway

10 Airway and Ventilation

Expanded Chapter Content

- Patient Positioning
- BVM Resuscitator
- Asthma and the Use of the Metered Dose Inhaler (MDI)

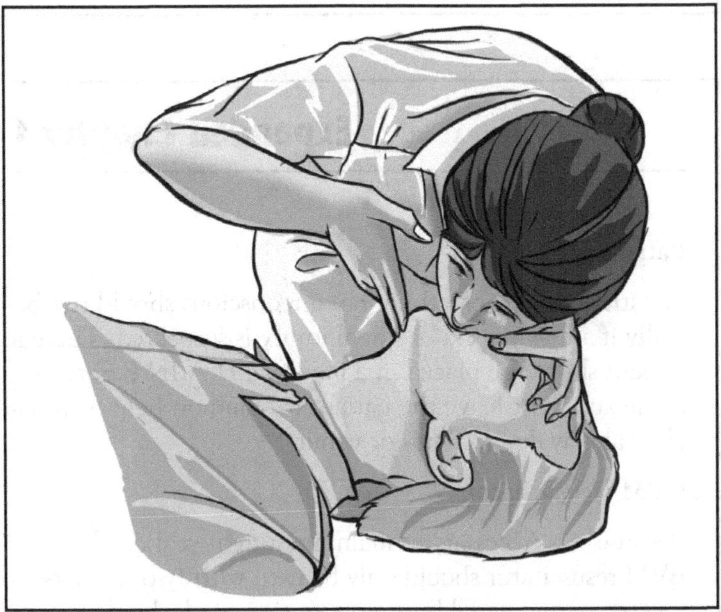

Chapter Significance

In Chapter 4, you learned the normal anatomy and physiology of various human body systems in order to understand disease conditions. In this chapter, various diseases and conditions related to the respiratory system are presented. It is important for the emergency medical responder to understand the pathophysiology of these diseases in order to provide the type of emergency care that the patient requires.

This chapter also discusses the signs and symptoms of ineffective breathing. As you learned, the emergency medical responder assesses a patient's breathing during the primary (initial) assessment. If during the primary assessment the EMR notices signs of ineffective breathing, he should immediately modify care in order to improve oxygenation. One simple technique to improve oxygen levels in an unconscious patient is to open the airway. The way in which the EMR opens the

CHECK • CALL • CARE

airway will depend on whether a head, neck, or spinal injury is suspected. If a patient is not breathing after the airway has been opened, the EMR will need to give artificial ventilations. When giving artificial ventilations, special situations such as vomiting; the presence of loose dentures; air in the stomach; head, neck, or spinal injury; or a stoma may be encountered by the emergency medical responder. These special situations may require changes in the way ventilations are delivered. An important tool for giving ventilations is the *bag-valve-mask* (BVM) resuscitator because it can deliver the highest concentrations of oxygen and is not as tiring to use as a resuscitation mask.

Expanded Chapter Content

Patient Positioning

A patient who is breathing but unconscious should not be moved from a face-up position, especially if a head, neck, or spinal injury is suspected. There are a few special situations in which the patient should be placed in a modified H.A.IN.E.S. recovery position and include if you are alone and must leave the patient to summon help or you are unable to maintain an open and clear airway due to fluids or vomit.

BVM Resuscitator

Because it is necessary to maintain a tight seal on the mask over a patient's nose and mouth, a BVM resuscitator should only be used with two rescuers to deliver artificial ventilations. If only one rescuer is available, a resuscitation mask should be used instead.

Sources

American Heart Association and the American National Red Cross (2010). Part 17: First aid: 2010 American Heart Association and American Red Cross Guidelines for First Aid. *Circulation* 122:S934-S946. http://circ.ahajournals.org/content/122/18_suppl_3/S394

Name: ______________________________ Date: ____________

Learning Activities

I. Multiple Choice

1. Which of the following actions would be appropriate for an emergency medical responder to take in caring for a patient who is hyperventilating due to anxiety?
   a. Encourage the patient to lie on her side to ease breathing.
   b. Administer oxygen if it is available and you are trained to use it.
   c. Ask the patient to breathe with you to slow down her breathing.
   d. Assist the patient in taking prescribed medications if you are authorized to do so.

2. The purpose of giving artificial ventilations is to
   a. Circulate oxygen-rich blood to all body cells
   b. Supplement the oxygen level in the air that the patient is breathing
   c. Supply the patient with oxygen, which is necessary for survival
   d. All of the above

3. An emergency medical responder would suspect that the patient is experiencing respiratory distress based on which of the following signs?
   a. Audible, high-pitched gurgling noises
   b. Complaints of "feeling tired"
   c. Sneezing with watery eyes
   d. Yellowish skin

4. A benefit of using a resuscitation mask to ventilate a patient is that it
   a. Decreases the risk of disease transmission
   b. Decreases the amount of air required to fully inflate the lungs
   c. Prevents the tongue from obstructing the airway
   d. All of the above

5. When you give two ventilations to a patient who is not breathing, you discover that the ventilations are not causing the patient's chest to rise. What should be your next step?
   a. Re-tilt the head and give two more ventilations.
   b. Check for a pulse.
   c. Administer two more ventilations but with greater force.
   d. Give five back blows, look in the mouth, and do a finger sweep if an object is seen.

6. In giving artificial ventilations to an unconscious patient, how much air should you breathe into the patient?
   a. Until you meet resistance
   b. Count to five in your head before taking your mouth off the mask
   c. Just until you notice the chest rising
   d. As much air as you are capable of delivering to the patient

7. After giving artificial ventilations for 2 minutes, the next step that an emergency medical responder should do is
   a. Call 9-1-1
   b. Switch with another trained rescuer
   c. Check for signs of life
   d. Begin CPR

8. You suspect that an unconscious patient has a spinal injury. You need to leave the patient to summon EMS. The patient is breathing and has a pulse. How should you position the patient?
   a. Leave the patient in a prone position.
   b. Leave the patient in a supine position.
   c. Place the patient in the most comfortable position.
   d. Place the patient in the H.A.IN.E.S recovery position.

9. To open a patient's airway using the jaw-thrust maneuver, an emergency medical responder should
   a. Tilt the patient's head back
   b. Maintain pressure on the patient's forehead
   c. Slide the fingers under the angles of the jawbone
   d. Lift the chin in an upward motion

10. An emergency medical responder knows that a patient's airway is open if
    a. The patient is unable to speak a full sentence
    b. You hear air coming out of the nose and mouth of the patient
    c. The patient is clutching his or her throat with one hand
    d. The chest does not rise and fall with ventilations

11. An unconscious adult was pulled from a swimming pool. When you open the airway to look, listen, and feel for breathing, the patient is taking infrequent gasps and has a weak pulse. What should you do next?
    a. Give two ventilations
    b. Check for severe bleeding
    c. Begin CPR
    d. Continue to monitor the patient's breathing

12. You are giving artificial ventilations to a 7-year-old boy with a resuscitation mask. How often should you give ventilations?
    a. Once every second
    b. Once every 2 seconds
    c. Once every 3 seconds
    d. Once every 5 seconds

13. You are positioned above a child's head and are using a resuscitation mask to give ventilations. After you position the mask, what should you do next?
    a. Seal the mask
    b. Blow into the mask
    c. Lower the mask over the mouth
    d. Open the airway

14. As you are giving ventilations to an adult in respiratory arrest, the patient vomits. What is the first action that an emergency medical responder should take in this situation?
   a. Clear the airway of the vomit immediately.
   b. Turn the patient as a unit onto his or her side.
   c. Use greater force when giving ventilations to bypass the vomit.
   d. Reposition the patient's head to reopen the airway.

15. Which of the following statements is correct in the use of a resuscitation mask?
   a. Cover the nose completely with the mask with the bottom edge at the upper lip.
   b. Place the broad end of the mask between the lower lip and chin.
   c. Blow into the mask for at least 2 seconds to give ventilations.
   d. Hold the mask at the one-way valve to seal it.

16. You and a fellow rescuer are giving ventilations using a bag-valve-mask resuscitator. One rescuer positions the mask over the patient's face. What should the second rescuer do?
   a. Squeeze the bag with both hands.
   b. Open the airway with the thumbs.
   c. Position the fingers behind the jawbone.
   d. Ensure that the mask is sealed.

II. Short Answer

1. Define the terms *respiratory distress* and *respiratory arrest*.

2. List five signs and symptoms of respiratory distress.

   1.

   2.

   3.

   4.

   5.

3. What happens during an asthma attack?

4. List three factors that can trigger an asthmatic attack.

   1.

   2.

   3.

5. Two types of medications that are often used to control and/or relieve an acute asthma attack are ______________________________ and ______________________________.

6. List three signs and symptoms of emphysema.

   1.

   2.

   3.

7. List three factors that can cause a person to hyperventilate.

   1.

   2.

   3.

8. List three signs and symptoms of hyperventilation.

   1.

   2.

   3.

9. Describe the general care an emergency medical responder would administer to a patient suffering from respiratory distress.

10. How does the patient get excess air in his stomach during ventilations?

11. Define the term *stoma*. What modifications need to be taken when giving artificial ventilations to a patient with a stoma?

12. What is the general "rule" to follow when giving artificial ventilations to a patient with dentures?

13. On an adult, artificial ventilations are performed at a rate of ______ ventilation every _______ seconds.

14. Brain damage can occur after _________ to _________minutes without oxygen.

15. Breathing for a patient who is not breathing is known as ________________________ ________________________.

16. The term which means "excess air in the stomach" is ______________________ ____________________.

17. The two techniques that can be used to open an airway are the ____________________ and the ________________________________.

18. For a patient with a suspected head, neck, or spinal injury, which technique should be used to open the airway?_____________________________

19. A disease characterized by a breakdown in the walls of the alveoli causing retention of carbon dioxide is called ___________________.

20. The medical term for a bluish discoloration of the skin and mucous membranes is ________________.

21. The medical term which refers to an insufficient amount of oxygen delivered to the cells is called ____________________.

22. Define the medical term *aspiration*.

23. Identify 4 characteristics of an effective resuscitation mask.

    1.

    2.

    3.

    4.

24. A child or an infant's heart usually stops due to a ______________________________, while an adult's heart stops due to ____________________.

III. True/False

_______ 1. A lone rescuer is unable to use a BVM resuscitator effectively.
_______ 2. Paradoxical breathing generally occurs following severe chest trauma.
_______ 3. A rale is an abnormal breath sound.
_______ 4. A complete absence of breathing is called apnea.
_______ 5. Stridor is caused by an airway obstruction.
_______ 6. A blood clot in the lungs is called acute pulmonary edema.
_______ 7. Emphysema is a type of chronic obstructive pulmonary disease.

IV. Scenarios

Scenario 1

When arriving at the scene of an accident, you notice that a man crashed his motorcycle into a utility pole, and is lying unconscious on the ground. His face is covered with blood and he does not appear to be breathing. (Questions 1–7 relate to Scenario 1.)

1. Which of the following techniques would be best to open this man's airway?
   a. Use the head-tilt, chin-lift.
   b. Pull his lower jaw forward by putting your thumb in his mouth and your fingers on the jaw.
   c. Lift his chin using a two-handed jaw-thrust.
   d. Turn his head to the side and clear any blood and foreign matter from his mouth.

2. After the emergency medical responder opens the man's airway, the patient is not breathing. Your first step is to administer two ventilations. What is your next step, assuming that your ventilations went in?
   a. Re-tilt the head and try to give two ventilations.
   b. Check for a pulse.
   c. Check for skin characteristics.
   d. Place the patient in a modified H.A.IN.E.S recovery position.

3. The man has a pulse but is not breathing. How often would you provide artificial ventilations to this patient?
   a. Once every second
   b. Once every 3 seconds
   c. Once every 5 seconds
   d. Once every minute

4. When administering artificial ventilations, the emergency medical responder understands that if the patient's airway is not adequately opened, the following condition(s) may occur.
   a. Air may enter the patient's stomach.
   b. Gastric distention can cause the patient to vomit.
   c. An adequate supply of oxygen may not reach the patient's lungs.
   d. All of the above conditions may occur

5. EMS arrives at the scene with a BVM resuscitator. The emergency medical responder should compress the bag of the BVM resuscitator until
   a. The patient's chest rises
   b. The bag is empty
   c. You meet airway resistance
   d. The bag reinflates

6. When using a BVM resuscitator to ventilate this patient, how often should you give ventilations?
   a. 3 breaths per minute
   b. 5 breaths per minute
   c. 12 breaths per minute
   d. 24 breaths per minute

7. Which statement about a bag-valve-mask (BVM) resuscitator is most accurate?
   a. Monitoring a patient for full exhalation is not required.
   b. A BVM must be used by two rescuers.
   c. BVMs are readily available to emergency medical responders.
   d. When used by a single rescuer, it is easy to coordinate with giving chest compressions.

Scenario 2
An 8-month-old infant was rescued from an apartment fire. During your primary (initial) assessment, you discover that the infant is unconscious and not breathing.
(Questions 1 and 2 refer to Scenario 2.)

1. What action will you take initially?
   a. Begin CPR
   b. Administer two slow ventilations
   c. Open the mouth and do a finger sweep
   d. Turn the infant face down and deliver five backblows

2. Where will you check for a presence of a pulse?
   a. At the carotid artery in the neck
   b. At the heart at the left nipple
   c. At the brachial artery in the upper arm
   d. At the radial artery in the wrist

Scenario 3

It is early morning and you are the lifeguard at a local pool. The pool is almost deserted. Two women were swimming earlier but they have finished their laps and headed toward the locker room. After a while, you notice one of the women leave. About 20 minutes later, you enter the locker room and see the other woman lying motionless on the wet floor next to a row of lockers. (Questions 1–3 refer to Scenario 3.)

1. After verifying that the scene is safe to enter, what is the first step to take in this situation?

2. The woman is unconscious, has a pulse but not breathing. What should you do next?

3. You need to leave the woman to activate EMS. How should you position her?

Scenario 4

At work, you are summoned to assist a fellow worker who is ill. When you arrive at the scene, you notice the person lying on the ground, having difficulty breathing. His skin is ashen and his respiratory rate is elevated. (Questions 1–3 refer to Scenario 4.)

1. Assuming the scene is safe, what questions should you ask the worker?

2. How would you position this patient to ease breathing?

3. Would you activate EMS for this patient? Provide a rationale for your answer.

Expanded Chapter Content

Asthma and the use of the metered dose inhaler (MDI)

Asthma is a disease that affects the small airways called the bronchioles. Exposure to an asthma trigger causes the following two effects: (1) narrowing of the bronchioles due to muscle spasms constricting the muscles around and inside the airways; and (2) increase in the production of mucus inside the bronchiole due to inflammation.

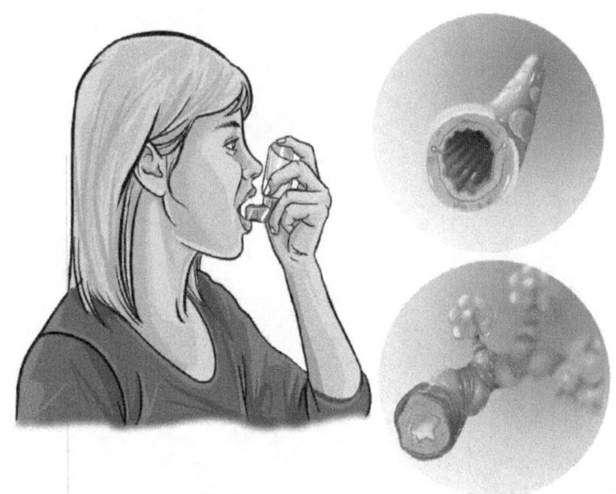

© hkannn, 2012. Used under license from Shutterstock, Inc.

The incidence of acute asthma is increasing, especially in urban settings. Many patients who have asthma take a prescribed bronchodilator medication, or *metered dose inhaler (MDI)*, that they self-administer. Emergency medical responders are not expected to make a diagnosis of asthma but may assist the patient to use the MDI if:

1. The patient states that he or she is having an asthma attack and has the prescribed medication in his or her possession.
2. The patient identifies the medication and is unable to administer it without assistance.

A spacer is often used between the *MDI* and the patient's mouth, especially in children and elderly individuals who have difficulty coordinating taking in a deep breath with depressing the inhaler canister.

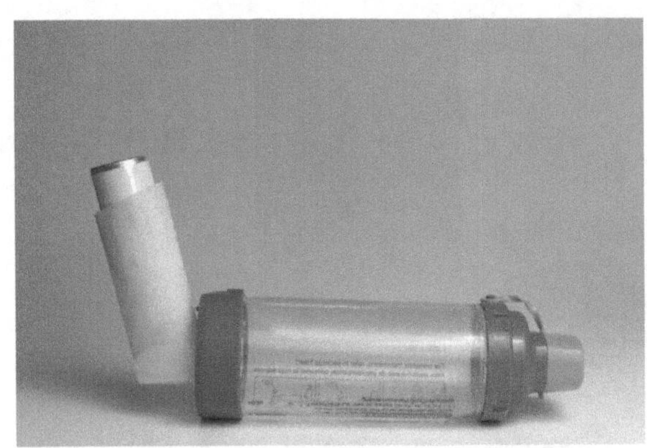

© Rob Byron, 2012. Used under license from Shutterstock, Inc.

11 Airway Management

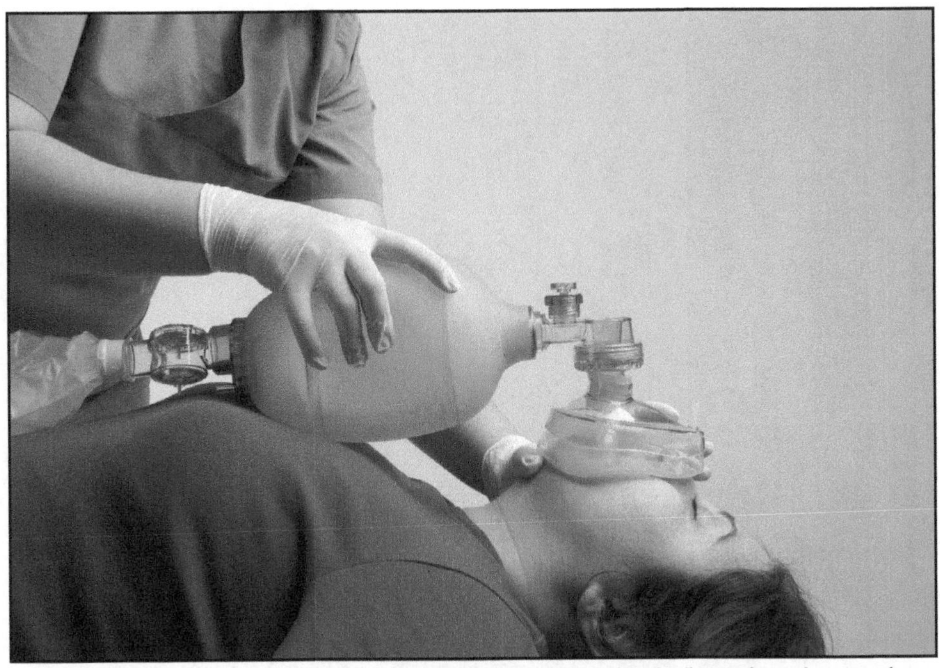

Chapter Significance

Managing breathing emergencies is one of the most important functions of an emergency medical responder. In Chapter 10, you learned how to assess and care for patients experiencing a breathing emergency such as respiratory distress or respiratory arrest, without the use of special equipment.

This chapter describes the various *airway adjuncts* that, when available, make it easier to maintain an open airway and support assisted ventilation. Sometimes an unconscious patient will vomit during artificial ventilations. While a finger sweep can remove large pieces of material, smaller particles remain which are difficult to remove. A manual or mechanical *suction device* can remove these smaller particles, saliva, or blood to prevent *aspiration*.

The two types of foreign body airway obstruction (FBAO) are examined in this chapter; the steps to take to clear an airway obstruction on a conscious and unconscious adult, child, and infant are also discussed.

CHECK · CALL · CARE

Name: ______________________________ Date: ______________

Learning Activities

I. Multiple Choice

1. To select the correct size for placement of an oropharyngeal airway (OPA), measure from the
   a. Tip of the nose to the earlobe
   b. Earlobe to the corner of the mouth
   c. Center of the mouth to the back of the throat
   d. Corner of the mouth to the Adam's apple

2. Suctioning can reduce the amount of oxygen reaching the lungs; therefore an adult patient should be suctioned for no more than ________ seconds at a time.
   a. 5
   b. 10
   c. 15
   d. 20

3. Which of the following steps would an emergency medical responder take to clear an obstructed airway in an obviously pregnant, conscious woman?
   a. Administer five backblows followed by five abdominal thrusts.
   b. Administer five backblows followed by five chest thrusts.
   c. Administer five backblows only.
   d. Administer five chest thrusts only.

4. Which of the following is least likely to cause a mechanical airway obstruction?
   a. Tongue
   b. Vomitus
   c. A chunk of food
   d. Loose dentures

5. The first step to take when deciding to insert an oral airway is
   a. Ensure that the patient is unconscious
   b. Select the proper airway size
   c. Open the patient's mouth
   d. Insert the airway toward the roof of the mouth

6. An oropharyngeal airway (OPA) should not be used for which of the following patients?
   a. A patient without a gag reflex
   b. A patient who is alert and talking
   c. A patient who is unconscious
   d. A patient with nasal trauma

7. When suctioning the mouth of a patient, which of the following actions is most appropriate for the emergency medical responder to take?
   a Measure the distance from the patient's earlobe to the tip of the nose.
   b. Suction for at least 20 seconds each time.
   c. Insert the suction tip as far back into the throat as possible.
   d. Apply suction while withdrawing the tip in a circular motion.

II. Short Answer

1. The acronym *OPA* stands for: ______________________________.

2. State the purpose of using airway adjuncts such as oral and nasal devices.

3. Give the contraindications to using an *oropharyngeal airway* (OPA).

4. What is the difference between a partial and complete airway obstruction?

5. Name the two types of airway obstructions and the causes of each one.

6. List the steps you would take to clear a foreign body airway obstruction in a conscious adult or child.

7. List the steps you would take to clear a foreign body airway obstruction in a conscious infant.

8. What care would an emergency medical responder provide to a patient who is choking, conscious, can speak, and cough?

9. Define the medical term *aspiration*.

10. Describe how a patient who is alone can self-administer abdominal thrusts.

11. After performing chest thrusts on an unconscious patient (adult, child, or infant) with a foreign body airway obstruction, a finger sweep is only done when ______________________________.

12. A finger sweep can only be performed on an ______________________________ patient.

13. The number of backblows and abdominal thrusts given to a conscious adult or child with a foreign body airway obstruction is ________.

14. The number of backblows and chest thrusts given to a conscious infant with a foreign body airway obstruction is __________.

15. The number of chest compressions given to an unconscious adult, child, or infant with a foreign body airway obstruction is ____________________.

III. True or False

______1. An oral airway cannot be used on conscious patients.
______2. The tip of the suction catheter should not be inserted past the base of the tongue.
______3. Insert an oral airway into the mouth with the tip pointed toward the floor of the mouth.

IV. Scenarios

Scenario 1

You are dispatched to a scene where an adult man is reported to be unconscious. Upon your arrival, the man is observed lying on the floor with a pool of vomit near his head. He does not appear to be breathing. (Questions 1–3 refer to Scenario 1.)

1. When you manually clear the vomit from the man's mouth, you should
   a. Use the cross finger technique to open the mouth
   b. Turn the man onto his side
   c. Lift the head and tilt the chin
   d. Pull the jaw forward to open the mouth

2. After removing the vomit, the patient fails to start breathing. You use your pocket mask to give artificial ventilations. The mask must be placed so
   a. The point of the mask rests on the chin
   b. One end of the mask rests on the forehead
   c. One end of the mask rests between the lower lip and the chin
   d. The mouth is covered but not the nose

3. Oxygen and additional breathing devices become available. Which breathing device would allow you to supply the highest concentration of oxygen to this nonbreathing patient?
   a. BVM resuscitator
   b. Nasal cannula
   c. Nonrebreather mask
   d. Resuscitation mask

Scenario 2

You are visiting a friend whose 9-month-old baby is sitting in a high chair eating cheerios. Suddenly the infant begins to turn blue and cannot cough, breathe, or cry. The mother is frantic and looks to you for help. (Questions 1–5 refer to Scenario 2.)

1. You quickly remove the infant from the high chair. What should you do next?
   a. Give the infant two slow breaths.
   b. Tilt the infant's head back and pull up on the jaw.
   c. Administer five chest thrusts using two fingers in the center of the chest.
   d. Give five backblows between the shoulder blades.

2. When administering backblows to an infant with a foreign body airway obstruction, the head should be
   a. Higher than the chest
   b. Turned to the side
   c. Lower than the chest
   d. Resting on your thigh

3. After repeating several cycles of five backblows followed by five chest thrusts, the infant becomes unconscious. What is the first action for the emergency medical responder to take?
   a. Activate EMS.
   b. Perform a finger sweep using the pinkie finger.
   c. Administer 30 chests thrusts.
   d. Attempt to give two ventilations.

4. To administer chest thrusts to a conscious choking infant, the emergency medical responder should use
   a. The heel of one hand
   b. The heel of two hands
   c. The pads of four fingers
   d. The pads of two or three fingers

5. After administering 30 chest thrusts, the emergency medical responder should
   a. Give two ventilations
   b. Check for a pulse in the brachial artery
   c. Give five backblows
   d. Perform a finger sweep if an object is seen

Scenario 3

You are having dinner at a restaurant when a woman seated nearby begins to choke. She is able to breathe and cough forcefully. (Questions 1–4 refer to Scenario 3.)

1. As an emergency medical responder, what is the first action that you should take?
   a. Stay with the woman and encourage her to keep coughing.
   b. Immediately deliver five backblows.
   c. Immediately administer five abdominal thrusts.
   d. Give her five chest thrusts.

2. Which of the following would you identify as the universal sign that a conscious person is choking and needs your help?
   a. Clutching the throat
   b. Coughing
   c. The inability to speak or cry
   d. Yelling out, "I'm choking."

3. To administer abdominal thrusts on a conscious, choking adult, where would you place your hands?
   a. At the navel
   b. Slightly above the navel
   c. Slightly below the navel
   d. Just below the xiphoid process

4. You are attempting to dislodge a foreign body from a conscious choking adult patient when the patient suddenly becomes unconscious. What is the next step that you should take?
   a. Attempt to reopen the patient's airway.
   b. Perform a finger sweep.
   c. Gently lower the patient to the ground.
   d. Open the mouth and give two ventilations.

12 Emergency Oxygen

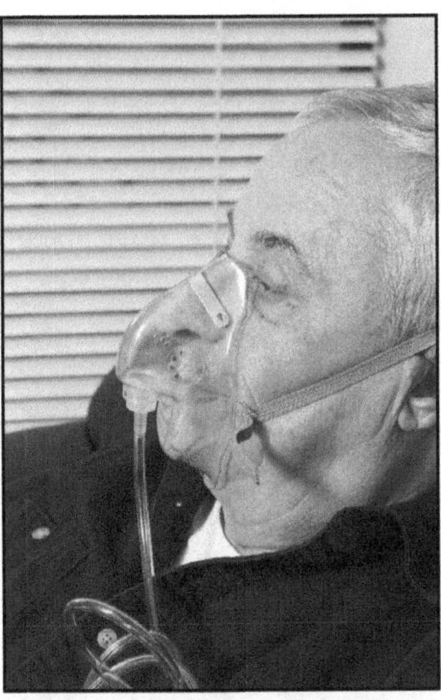

© fred goldstein, 2011. Used under license from Shutterstock, Inc.

Chapter Significance

Oxygen is essential for survival. A patient who is experiencing respiratory distress is not getting enough oxygen into the lungs for transport to all the cells in the body through the circulatory system. The patient with inadequate oxygenation will suffer from *hypoxia* causing increased respiratory distress and a bluish discoloration of the skin and nail beds (*cyanosis*). As you will learn in Chapter 13, a patient with coronary heart disease in which the coronary arteries are blocked by fatty plaques (*atherosclerosis*) will experience chest pain due to inadequate oxygenation of the heart muscle (*ischemia*). Being trained to administer oxygen in these situations will help the patient's respiratory distress and may alleviate their symptoms.

Oxygen can be delivered through a variety of devices including a mask with an oxygen inlet, nasal cannula, non-rebreather mask, and a bag-valve-mask (BVM) resuscitator. It is important for the emergency medical responder to understand the nature of the patient's problem and select the appropriate device to deliver supplemental oxygen.

CHECK ▪ CALL ▪ CARE

Name: ______________________ Date: __________

Learning Activities

I. Multiple Choice

1. Emergency oxygen should be administered to which of the following patients?
   a. An adult breathing less than 12 or more than 20 breaths per minute
   b. A child breathing less than 15 or more than 30 breaths per minute
   c. An infant breathing less than 25 or more than 50 breaths per minute
   d. All of the above

2. An oxygen delivery system which gives the emergency medical responder flexibility in adjusting the flow of oxygen being delivered to a patient is called a
   a. Fixed flow rate
   b. Pressure regulator
   c. Variable flow rate
   d. Flowmeter

3. Which type of oxygen delivery system can be used on a patient who is breathing?
   a. Nasal cannula
   b. BVM resuscitator
   c. Non-rebreather mask
   d. All of the above

4. Oxygen concentrations of 90% and above are achieved using which of the following types of oxygen delivery systems?
   a. Mask
   b. Non-rebreather mask
   c. BVM resuscitator
   d. Nasal cannula

5. You are preparing to administer emergency oxygen to a patient via a variable-flow-rate system. What is the first step that an emergency medical responder should take?
   a. Clear the valve.
   b. Attach the regulator.
   c. Check the cylinder label and markings.
   d. Open the cylinder counterclockwise one full turn.

6. When using emergency oxygen, which of the following statements is most appropriate to remember?
   a. The valve or regulator should be used to carry the cylinder.
   b. Oxygen cylinders should stand in an upright position on a flat surface.
   c. Using grease or oil to clean the regulator could lead to an explosion.
   d. Cylinders should be dragged but not rolled.

7. Which statement best reflects a variable-flow-rate system?
   a. The system is already preassembled.
   b. The flow rate has a high or low setting.
   c. The flow rate can be adjusted for use with various oxygen delivery devices.
   d. It is less practical than other types of systems.

8. You are preparing to administer oxygen to a patient with a nasal injury. Of the following oxygen delivery devices, which one is least appropriate to use on this patient?
   a. Non-rebreather mask
   b. Nasal Cannula
   c. Resuscitation mask
   d. Bag-valve-mask resuscitator

II. Short Answer

1. Safety is a major concern in the preparation and use of emergency oxygen. List the 9 safety precautions that should be followed in the administration of oxygen.

   1.

   2.

   3.

   4.

   5.

   6.

   7.

   8.

   9.

2. A decreased amount of oxygen in the blood is called____________________.

3. The air that a person normally breathes in contains about __________% oxygen; the percent of oxygen in exhaled air is about __________%.

4. The amount of oxygen administered to a patient through a resuscitation mask is about ________%.

5. A fixed flow rate oxygen system is preset to administer oxygen at the flow rate of __________ liters per minute (LPM).

6. If the pressure gauge on an oxygen cylinder reads 200 pounds per square inch (psi), what should the emergency medical responder do?

Unit 4

Circulation

13 Circulation and Cardiac Emergencies

EXPANDED CHAPTER CONTENT

- Risk Factors for Heart Disease
- Use of an AED
- AED and CPR
- Witnessed Sudden Collapse of an Adult
- Two Rescuer CPR—Child and Infant

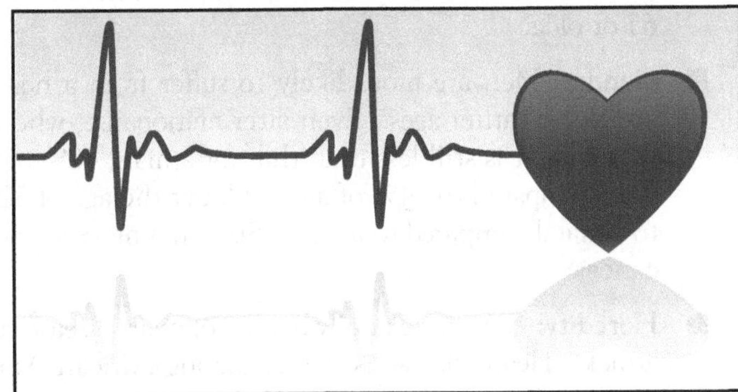

Chapter Significance

Heart disease is the number one cause of death for men and women in the United States, claiming approximately 1 million lives annually. Every 33 seconds, someone in the United States dies from cardiovascular disease. By 2020, heart disease will be the leading cause of death throughout the world. In 2008, the total cost of cardiovascular disease in the United States (including coronary heart disease, hypertensive disease, heart failure, and stroke) was estimated at $448.5 billion! While these are staggering statistics, they underscore the magnitude of the disease and the overwhelming financial burden on the health care system.

The incidence of heart disease increases with advancing age. The development of heart disease is multifactorial—the more risk factors one has, the higher the incidence of heart disease. In this chapter, you will study the risk factors for the development of heart disease and learn how to decrease those risk factors. You will also learn how to save a patient's life through CPR and the use of an AED. This knowledge is especially critical to an adult patient who is likely to suffer from a cardiac emergency.

CHECK ▪ CALL ▪ CARE

Risk Factors for Heart Disease

Many risk factors have been identified as producing significant threats associated with heart disease. These risk factors are classified into two categories: modifiable and nonmodifiable. There are also contributing risk factors whose significance and prevalence in the risk for heart disease have not been precisely determined.

Nonmodifiable risk factors:

- **Increasing Age:** The risk of death from coronary heart disease increases dramatically after the age of 65. Statistics show that 83% of individuals who die as a result of coronary heart disease are age 65 or older.
- **Gender:** Men are more likely to suffer from a heart attack than women; they also have heart attacks at earlier ages. Even after menopause, when a woman's risk for death from heart attacks increases, it is still less than that for a man; 42% of women who have heart attacks die within 1 year, compared to 24% of men. Under the age of 50, a heart attack in a woman is twice as likely to be fatal compared to a man. Six times more women die from heart disease than die from breast cancer.
- **Heredity:** A positive family history of heart disease can increase the risk of a person having a heart attack. Heart disease is higher among African Americans, American Indians, Alaska Natives, Asian or Pacific Islanders, and Hispanics. Genetic factors are likely to play some role in the development of high blood pressure, heart disease, and other vascular conditions. However, it is also likely that people with a family history of heart disease share common environments and risk factors that jeopardize their heart health.

Modifiable risk factors:

- **Smoking:** The risk for developing coronary heart disease in smokers is two to three times higher than in nonsmokers. People who smoke cigars and pipes have a higher risk of death from coronary heart disease but the risk is smaller than from cigarette smoking. Cigarette smoking promotes atherosclerosis and increases the levels of blood clotting factors, such as fibrinogen. Nicotine also raises blood pressure, and carbon monoxide reduces the amount of oxygen that blood can carry. Exposure to secondhand smoke can also raise the risk of heart disease for nonsmokers.
- **High cholesterol levels:** To understand the cholesterol numbers, one needs to look at the total cholesterol level (which should be less than 200) as well as the levels of HDL (high density lipoprotein, or good cholesterol) and LDL (low density lipoprotein, or bad cholesterol). A good level of HDL cholesterol is at least 60 mg/dL; levels between 40 and 60 are considered OK. An optimal level of LDL cholesterol is under 100 mg/dL. To find your cholesterol ratio, divide your total cholesterol number by your HDL, or good, cholesterol number. For example, if your total cholesterol number is 200 and your good cholesterol is 50, your total cholesterol ratio is 4:1. According to the American Heart Association, you should keep your cholesterol ratio at or below 5:1. The ideal cholesterol ratio is about 3.5:1. Low levels of HDL or high levels of LDL increase one's risk for coronary heart disease. Cholesterol levels can be lowered through dietary modifications, exercise, and medication.
- **High blood pressure (hypertension):** An elevated blood pressure increases the workload of the heart, causing the heart muscle to thicken and become stiffer. Blood pressure can be lowered through medications, dietary modifications (reduced salt), and exercise.

- **Physical inactivity:** A sedentary lifestyle can lead to obesity, a risk factor for coronary heart disease. Regular exercise can lower blood pressure, reduce blood cholesterol and blood sugar levels (causing diabetes), improve one's emotional outlook, and reduce stress.
- **Obesity:** Obesity is excess body fat. Excess weight places an added strain on the heart, increasing its workload. Most individuals who are obese also have high cholesterol levels, high blood pressure, and high blood sugar levels. Obesity is linked to higher LDL (bad) cholesterol and triglyceride (another form of fat in the blood) levels and to lower HDL (good) cholesterol, high blood pressure, and diabetes. A modest weight loss of just 10 pounds can lower one's risk for coronary heart disease.
- **Diabetes mellitus:** Diabetes mellitus destroys arteries in major organs causing kidney failure (leading to dialysis), damage to the retina (retinopathy) causing blindness, and nervous system disease (neuropathy) causing numbness and tingling in the fingers and toes (and possible loss of limbs). Research has demonstrated that diabetes also affects the coronary arteries, greatly increasing the risk for coronary heart disease and heart attack. Diabetes can be controlled with diet, exercise, and medication.
- **Alcohol:** Increased alcohol use can cause obesity, raise blood pressure, and cause coronary heart disease by damaging the heart muscle. Excessive alcohol use also increases blood levels of triglycerides which contributes to atherosclerosis.

Contributing risk factors:

- **Stress:** You have probably heard of a "type A personality," the person who has a very stressful job, overreacts to problems, yells, has trouble sleeping, and drinks a lot of coffee. Individuals who experience a tremendous amount of stress in their daily lives, without an outlet for that stress, may experience coronary heart disease in the form of a heart attack. Stress is often associated with leading a sedentary lifestyle, smoking, obesity, and poor eating habits, all risk factors for coronary heart disease.

Automated External Defibrillator (AED)

An ***automated external defibrillator (AED)*** is an external device capable of analyzing the patient's heart rhythm and delivering a shock to the heart to reverse a life-threatening rhythm. To defibrillate is to administer a shock to the heart. The availability and proper use of a defibrillator within minutes of sudden cardiac arrest can greatly increase a patient's chance for survival. The combination of early CPR coupled with defibrillation has been shown to produce the highest survival rates for an adult suffering from a sudden cardiac arrest. Many patients experience a chaotic heart rhythm (ventricular fibrillation or ventricular tachycardia) following a heart attack. Chaotic heart rhythms can only be reversed with an AED.

Rationale for early defibrillation:

1. The most frequent initial rhythm in sudden cardiac arrest is ventricular fibrillation.
2. The most effective treatment for ventricular fibrillation is defibrillation.
3. The probability of successful defibrillation decreases rapidly over time.
4. Ventricular fibrillation tends to convert to ***asystole*** ("flat line") within a few minutes.

Operation of the AED—adult, child, infant:

1. Confirm cardiac arrest. Check for consciousness, breathing, and signs of life for no more than 10 seconds.
2. Turn on the AED.
3. Wipe the patient's chest dry. If necessary, shave the areas where the pads are to be placed. The adhesive pads must be applied to the bare chest. Follow the instruction on the pads: place one pad over the patient's right shoulder, and place the second pad on the left side of the patient's chest under the breast.
   - For a child (ages 1–8) or infant (0–1 year), pediatric pads must be used. One pad is placed in the center of the child/infant's chest, and the second pad is placed in the center of the child/infant's back.

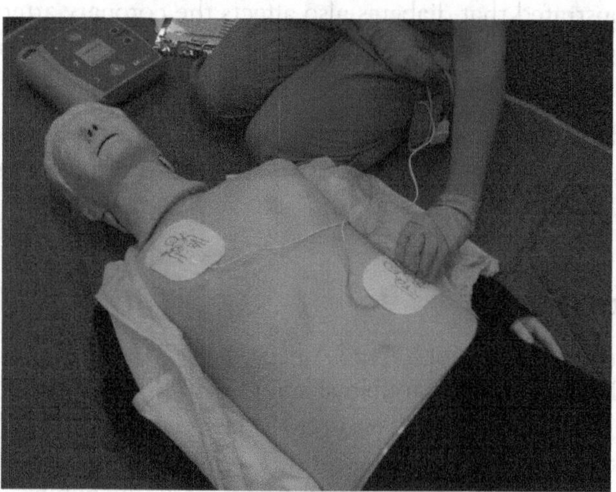

Figure 13.1
For an adult, apply one pad on the patient's right shoulder area, and apply the second pad on the patient's left chest area, just under the breast.

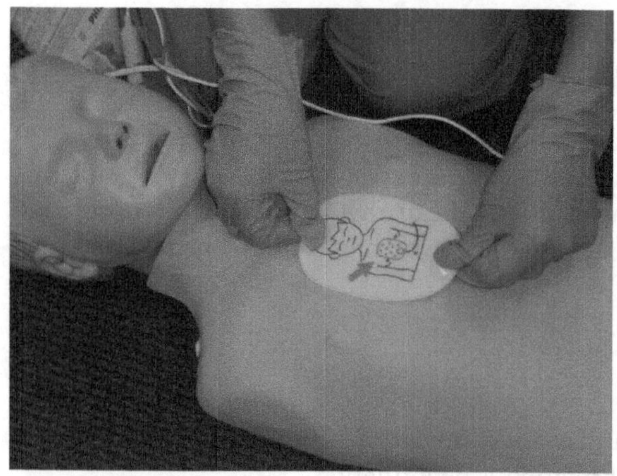

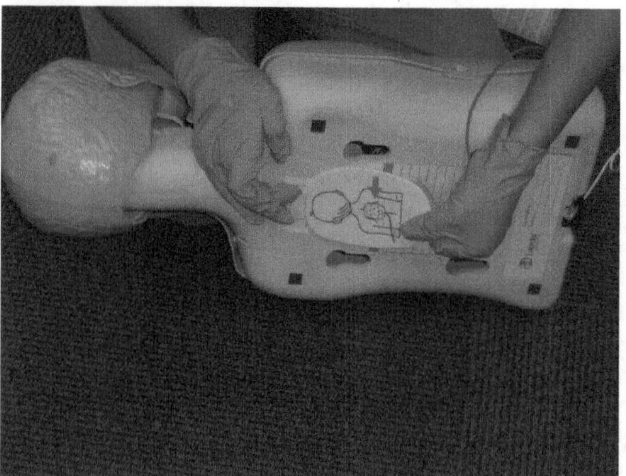

Figure 13.2
Notice that pediatric AED pads are placed in the center of the child/infant's chest and on the center of the back. The electric current flows front to back (anterior to posterior) rather than diagonally across the heart, as in an adult. This is the preferred placement because a child or infant has a small chest area; placement of pads on the right shoulder and under the left breast area may cause the pads to touch each other.

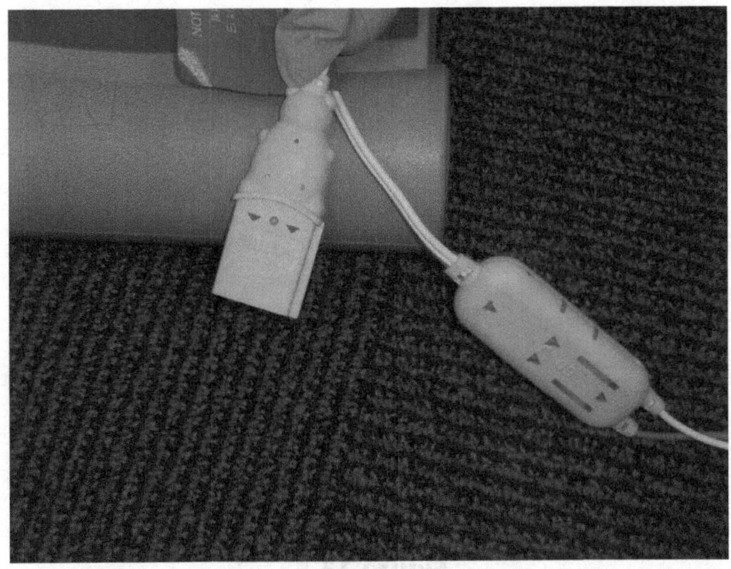

Figure 13.3
This is a pediatric AED cable. Notice that the connector has a "teddy bear" shape on the end and that there is an extra yellow "bump" in the cable. If you look closely, you will see "50 J" imprinted on it. The electrical output is reduced to 50 joules at this point before it is delivered to a pediatric patient.

4. Plug the connector into the AED.
   - **Child/infant:** You must use a special AED that can deliver lower joules. If this type of AED is not available, then a pediatric cable must be used to reduce the electrical output to 50 joules.
5. Allow the AED to analyze the heart rhythm. Stop CPR and do not touch the patient while the machine is analyzing the heart rhythm. If the AED gives the "no shock advised" message, begin CPR for 2 minutes. After 2 minutes, the AED will reanalyze the heart rhythm. If no shock is advised, continue CPR for another 2 minutes. If at any time you notice signs of life, stop CPR and monitor the ABCs.
6. If the AED gives the "shock advised" message, ensure that no one, including yourself, is touching the patient and that no hazards are present (standing puddles of water, flammable materials). Deliver the shock and resume CPR for 2 minutes. After 2 minutes, the AED will reanalyze the heart rhythm (stop CPR). If a shock is advised, make sure no one is touching the patient, deliver the shock, and continue CPR for an additional 2 minutes if needed.

In the event that a rescuer is alone and an AED is immediately available, the recommended sequence is to verify unresponsiveness, check for signs of life, then activate 9-1-1. If there is no pulse, the rescuer should turn on the AED, wipe the chest and shave if necessary, apply the pads, and proceed with analysis and a shock, if indicated. An AED can only be applied to a pulseless patient.

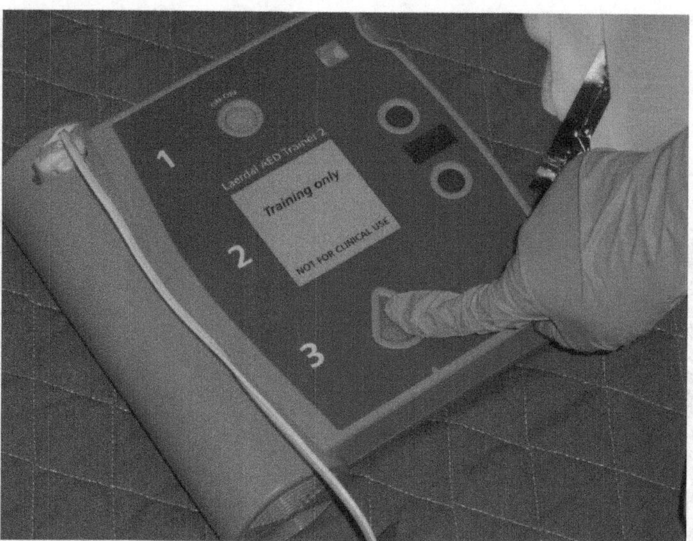

Figure 13.4
Prior to depressing the shock button, make sure that no one, including the operator, is touching the patient. On a real AED, the operator will be able to see the heart's electrical activity in the square marked "training only." This information guides the treatment plan by the emergency medical responder and EMS.

Expanded Chapter Content

Expanded Chapter Content: AED and CPR
If CPR is in progress when an AED becomes available, do not stop CPR while the AED is readied for use. The machine should be turned on, the patient's chest wiped dry, the pads applied, and the connector plugged in BEFORE CPR is stopped. In this situation, CPR must be stopped for the following reasons: The AED is analyzing the heart rhythm, the AED is preparing to deliver a shock to the heart, or the patient shows signs of life.

Two shockable rhythms:

1. **Ventricular fibrillation:** the heart is quivering and no blood is being pumped out of the heart; the patient will have no pulse. This is a totally disorganized, chaotic, electrical activity resulting in the inability of the heart to pump blood.
2. **Ventricular tachycardia:** the ventricles (lower chambers) are beating rapidly. The pulse will either be very weak or absent. Due to the rapid beating of the heart, the ventricles are not able to fill with blood, causing cardiac output to be decreased.

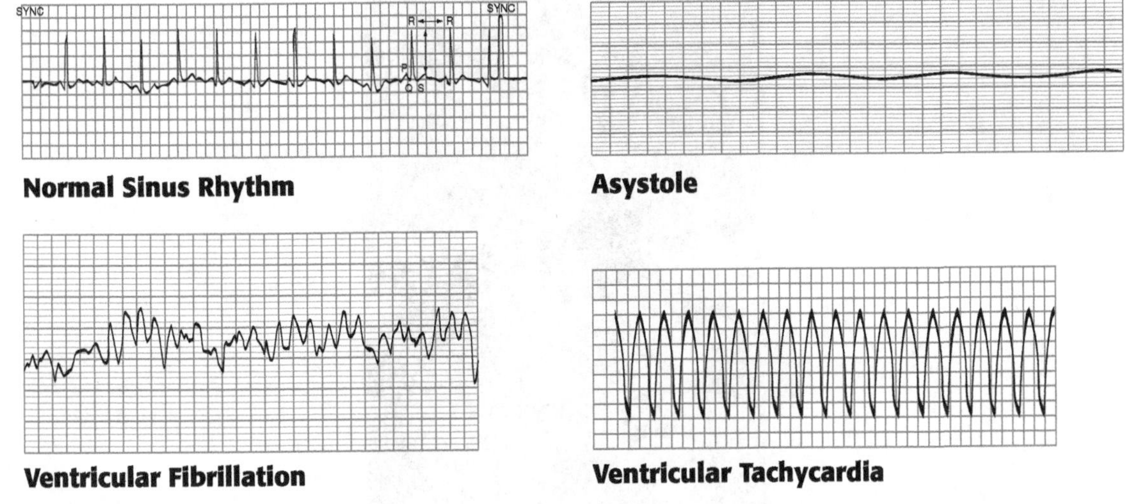

TOP LEFT: *Normal Sinus Rhythm*—the normal rhythm of the heart

TOP RIGHT: *Asystole*—also known as a "flatline." The heart is not beating. This is not a shockable rhythm, and CPR is needed.

BOTTOM LEFT: *Ventricular Fibrillation (V-fib)*—no pulse because the heart is "quivering," not beating. This is a shockable rhythm. Usually converts to asystole after a few minutes.

BOTTOM RIGHT: *Ventricular Tachycardia (V-tach)*—if felt, a pulse will be weak. Ventricular tachycardia can progress into ventricular fibrillation. This is a shockable rhythm.

Most AEDs are set to deliver a preset electrical output (joules). The AED can deliver only one shock before it resets itself. After two minutes of CPR, the AED will reanalyze the patient's heart rhythm and give a "shock advised" or a "no shock advised" message. Most adults suffer cardiac arrest and a life-threatening arrhythmia due to a cardiac problem; an AED can reverse a life-threatening arrhythmia. CPR cannot reverse ventricular fibrillation or ventricular tachycardia. An AED is rarely used on a child or infant because the heart stops due to a respiratory problem. Once the breathing problem is corrected, the heart will restart. Look for the sign that indicates the presence of an AED. They are often found in gymnasiums, schools, airports, malls, and stores (Figure 13.5).

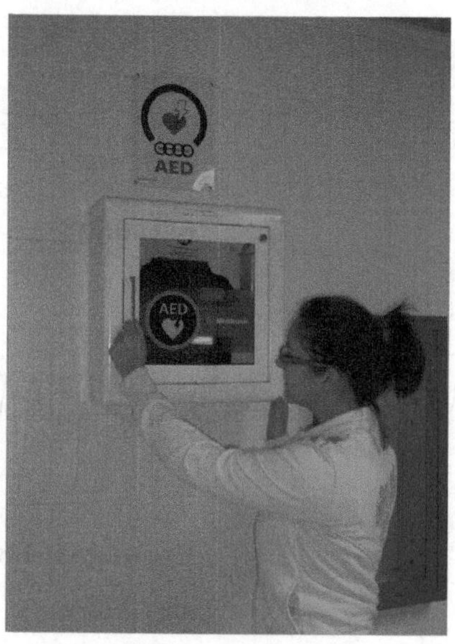

Figure 13.5
An AED can be found in many locations.

Sources

www.americanheart.org Heart Disease & Stroke Statistics

American Heart Association and the American National Red Cross (2010). Part 17: First Aid: 2010 American Heart Association and American Red Cross Guidelines for First Aid. *Circulation* 112: S934-S946. www.circulationaha.org

http://www.cdc.gov/nchs/FASTATS/heart.htm

http://www.cdc.gov/heartdisease/facts.htm

http://www.the heartfoundation.org/heart-disease-facts/heart-disease-statistics/

Name: ______________________ Date: ____________

Learning Activities

I. Multiple Choice

1. The purpose of cardiopulmonary resuscitation (CPR) is to
   a. Keep the brain supplied with oxygen until the heart starts beating
   b. Prevent clinical death from occurring
   c. Restart the heartbeat and breathing in a patient
   d. All of the above

2. The most common cause of cardiac emergencies in children is
   a. Poisoning
   b. Electrocution
   c. Trauma to the head
   d. Respiratory problems

3. What should an emergency medical responder do if the patient shows signs of life while performing CPR?
   a. Instruct a bystander to transport her and the patient to the nearest hospital.
   b. Perform artificial ventilations only until EMS arrives.
   c. Perform a physical examination and SAMPLE history
   d. Leave the patient on his back and perform an ongoing assessment every 5 minutes.

4. During two-rescuer adult CPR, the rescuer at the patient's head should give breaths and
   a. Count the number of chest compressions out loud
   b. Periodically check for the carotid pulse
   c. Stop the compressions every 2 minutes to check for signs of life
   d. All of the above

5. The most well-known sign of a heart attack is
   a. Difficulty breathing
   b. Sweating
   c. Nausea
   d. Persistent chest pain

6. How should a patient who may be experiencing a heart attack be positioned?
   a. The most comfortable position for the patient
   b. Sitting or semi-sitting in a chair
   c. Lying on the left side
   d. Lying on the back with the legs elevated

7. High blood pressure can be controlled by
   a. Becoming more active
   b. Losing weight
   c. Taking medication
   d. All of the above

8. To deliver effective chest compressions on an adult in cardiac arrest, your hands should be placed
   a. Over the xiphoid process
   b. Over the lower half of the breastbone
   c. On the middle of the breastbone
   d. Just above the nipple line

9. Cardiac arrest is identified by the
   a. Absence of breathing
   b. Absence of movement
   c. Absence of a pulse
   d. Dilation of the pupils

10. To deliver chest compressions on a child, you would use the
    a. Heel of one hand
    b. Pads of two fingers
    c. Heel of two hands
    d. Pads of three fingers

11. On an adult, the chest should be compressed at a depth of ______inches during CPR.
    a. 1 ½
    b. about 2
    c. at least 2
    d. 3

12. The cycle of two-rescuer CPR in an infant is
    a. 30 compressions and 2 ventilations
    b. 15 compressions and 2 ventilations
    c. 5 compressions and 1 ventilation
    d. 5 compressions and 2 ventilations

13. To give effective chest compressions to an infant in cardiac arrest, the chest must be depressed
    a. ½ inch
    b. 1 inch
    c. 1 ½ inches
    d. 2 inches

14. The cycle of compressions and ventilations given by two rescuers to an adult in cardiac arrest is
    a. 30 compresions and 2 ventilations
    b. 30 compressions and 1 ventilation
    c. 15 compressions and 2 ventilations
    d. 15 compressions and 1 ventilation

15. The correct hand position for CPR in an infant is
    a. One hand on the forehead and two or three fingers on the sternum just below the nipple line
    b. One hand on the forehead and two or three fingers on the sternum just above the nipple line
    c. One hand on the forehead and two or three fingers on the sternum on the xiphoid process
    d. One hand on the forehead and the pads of two or three fingers directly in the center of the chest, across from the nipple line

16. While preparing the AED for use, you notice that the patient has a medication patch on his chest. Which of the following actions would be most appropriate for the emergency medical responder to take?
    a. Wipe the chest dry avoiding the area where the medication patch is applied.
    b. Place one pad on the patient's back and the second patch on the chest at least 4 inches away from the medication patch.
    c. Leave the medication patch in place and apply the pads as you normally would.
    d. With a gloved hand, remove the medication patch and wipe the skin.

17. You are about the apply the AED pads to an adult female patient's chest when you notice that she has several body piercings with jewelry. What would be the most appropriate action for the emergency medical responder to take in this situation?
    a. Apply the pads to the chest, avoiding the jewelry.
    b. Remove the body piercings prior to applying the pads.
    c. Wipe the chest dry with alcohol, including the jewelry.
    d. Apply the pads as you normally would, even if the pad is over the body piercing.

18. You are performing CPR alone when a second rescuer arrives to help. What should the second rescuer do first?
    a. Check to see whether EMS has been activated.
    b. Call for a change in position to assist with CPR.
    c. Tell the first rescuer to stop CPR so the patient can be assessed.
    d. Begin giving ventilations to the patient.

19. The cycle of CPR given to a 6-year-old is
    a. 15 compressions and 1 ventilation
    b. 15 compressions and 2 ventilations
    c. 30 compressions and 2 ventilations
    d. 30 compressions and 1 ventilation

20. What action should an emergency medical responder take if the AED gives a "no shock advised" message?
    a. Turn off the AED for 5 seconds, then turn it back on to allow the machine to reanalyze the heart rhythm.
    b. Monitor the patient's airway and breathing.
    c. Readjust the pad placement on the patient's chest.
    d. Perform CPR for 2 minutes.

21. After applying the AED pads to a patient's chest and plugging in the pads connector, the next step would be to
    a. Push the "analyze' button
    b. Press the "shock" button
    c. Tell everyone to stand clear
    d. Turn on the AED

22. The most important action taken by the emergency medical responder to ensure that chest compressions are effective is to
    a. Place the hands at the upper part of the chest, above the nipple line
    b. Allow the chest to fully recoil between compressions
    c. Position the patient on a soft, flat surface
    d. Compress the chest to a shallow depth

23. The first step in the Cardiac Chain of Survival is
    a. Early defibrillation
    b. Early CPR
    c. Early recognition and access to the EMS system
    d. Early more advanced medical care

24. You are providing care to a patient with chest pain who may be having a heart attack. Your first action would be to
    a. Summom EMS
    b. Loosen any tight clothing
    c. Administer two baby aspirin tablets
    d. Monitor the patient's vital signs

25. The target number of chest compressions to give in 1 minute to an adult, child, or infant is
    a. 60
    b. 80
    c. 100
    d. 120

26. Where should an emergency medical responder place the AED pads on an infant or a child?
    a. One pad on the patient's right upper shoulder and one pad on the chest, just under the left breast
    b. One pad on the center of the chest and one pad on the center of the back
    c. One pad on the center of the chest and one pad over the left thigh
    d. One pad on the patient's left upper shoulder and one pad on the chest, just under the right breast

27. The most common rhythm associated with sudden cardiac arrest is
    a. Ventricular tachycardia
    b. Atrial fibrillation
    c. Ventricular fibrillation
    d. Sinus rhythm

II. Short Answer

1. What is meant by the medical term *atherosclerosis*?

2. What is the difference between *angina pectoris* and a *heart attack*?

3. List three modifiable and three nonmodifiable risk factors for cardiovascular disease.

   Modifiable

   1.

   2.

   3.

   Nonmodifiable

   1.

   2.

   3.

4. List five signs and symptoms of a heart attack.

   1.

   2.

   3.

   4.

   5.

5. Another term used to denote a heart attack is ______________________.

6. List the eight steps to take in providing care to a patient with a cardiac emergency.

   1.

   2.

   3.

   4.

   5.

   6.

   7.

   8.

7. Prior to the administration of aspirin to a patient with chest pain, what questions should the emergency medical responder ask the patient?

8. What does CPR stand for, and what is its purpose?

9. What is the cycle of compressions and ventilations when performing one-rescuer CPR on an infant, child, and adult?

10. How does the performance of CPR differ when there is one rescuer versus two rescuers?

11. List seven circumstances in which it is acceptable to stop CPR.

    1.

    2.

    3.

    4.

    5.

    6.

    7.

12. Name the four links in the *Cardiac Chain of Survival*.

13. What does the abbreviation *AED* stand for?

14. Prior to applying an AED on a patient, the emergency medical responder must verify that the patient is ____________________.

15. Name the two shockable heart rhythms the AED is programmed to recognize.

16. Where are the AED pads placed on an adult patient? On a child or infant?

17. What action should an emergency medical responder take if the AED gives a "shock advised" message?

18. Why is it important to stand clear of the patient before delivering a shock?

III. True or False

_______ 1. After doing 2 minutes of CPR on an infant, you should check the brachial pulse for no more than 10 seconds.

_______ 2. Brief, mild chest pain is usually a symptom of angina pectoris.

_______ 3. Immediate activation of 9-1-1 is important for a patient in cardiac arrest.

_______ 4. It can be difficult to find the correct hand position for chest compressions on an obese person because fat accumulates over the sternum.

_______ 5. CPR should be stopped completely if the patient vomits.

_______ 6. For a patient complaining of chest pain, an emergency medical responder should help the patient take his or her prescribed medication if authorized to do so.

_______ 7. The carotid pulse may be difficult to feel, even with effective chest compressions, if a patient has lost a significant amount of blood.

_______ 8. Exercising at least three times per week has been shown to reduce the risk of cardiovascular disease.

_______ 9. If an emergency medical responder is trained, the administration of oxygen is appropriate emergency care for a patient experiencing chest pain or discomfort.

IV. Crossword Puzzle

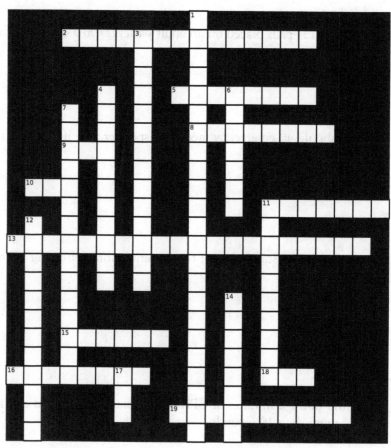

Across

2 A brief episode of chest pain that subsides with rest or medication.
5 The name of the artery found in the upper arm.
8 The name of the arteries that supply the heart muscle with oxygen-rich blood.
9 The abbreviation for good cholesterol.
10 The abbreviation for giving a cycle of chest compressions and ventilations.
11 A medication used to thin the blood in a person having chest pain.
13 Causes death of heart muscle.
15 The heart's electrical activity begins here, also known as the pacemaker of the heart.
16 A condition of no electrical activity in the heart, "flatline".
18 The abbreviation for the machine that delivers an electric shock to the heart.
19 The type of risk factors for heart disease that can be controlled or treated.

Down

1 A totally disorganized, chaotic heart rhythm.
3 The name of a small pill placed under the tongue in a patient experiencing chest pain.
4 The fatty substance that builds up in an artery.
6 The name of the artery found in the neck.
7 Narrowing and hardening of coronary arteries due to build up of cholesterol.
11 Irregular heart rhythm.
12 The medical term for high blood pressure.
14 Reduced blood flow to the heart muscle.
17 The abbreviation for bad cholesterol.

V. Scenarios

Scenario 1

You are called to the scene of an emergency where a 6-year-old child has just been pulled from a swimming pool after being submerged for several minutes. The child is unconscious, has no signs of life, and you feel no pulse. (Questions 1–4 refer to Scenario 1.)

True or False

_______ 1. In this situation, it is best to administer ventilations only.
_______ 2. The sternum of the child should be depressed 1½ inches with each chest compression.
_______ 3. The target number of chest compressions that should be given to this child is 100 per minute.

4. In order to deliver chest compressions to this child, you would use the
   a. Heel of one hand
   b. Heel of two hands
   c. Pads of two fingers
   d. Encircling chest technique

Scenario 2

During an office meeting, a co-worker who is giving a presentation suddenly stops, complaining of chest pain and shortness of breath. She is very pale and sweating. (Questions 1–4 refer to Scenario 2.)

1. What is the first step that you would take in caring for this patient?
   a. Have her stop the presentation and sit down.
   b. Activate 9-1-1.
   c. Turn on a fan and direct it on the patient.
   d. Have her lie on the floor and elevate her legs 12 inches.

2. Describe five actions you would take for this patient while waiting for advanced medical personnel to arrive.

3. If the patient is experiencing a heart attack, why is it very important for EMS to arrive quickly?

4. Based on these signs and symptoms, do you believe that the woman may be experiencing a heart attack? Provide rationale for your answer.

Scenario 3

In the early morning, you respond to a call dispatched as a "heart attack." You find an elderly man lying motionless on the floor. His wife tells you that he had been feeling ill for several hours and had vomited. She says that he emerged from the bathroom clutching his chest and in apparent pain, and suddenly collapsed on the floor. (Questions 1–3 refer to Scenario 3.)

1. During your initial assessment, **identify the signs and symptoms from the scenario** which suggest that the victim had a heart attack.

2. List three **additional** signs or symptoms of a heart attack.

3. Since it is safe to approach the victim, what is the **first** action you would take?

V. Web-Based Exercise (Extra Credit Assignment)

AED laws vary from state to state. Go to the website www.cprinstructor.com/legal.htm. Then click on "EMS, CPR, AED Legal Database-case law." From the list of states, select one state and answer the following questions about the AED law for that state.

Name of state selected____.

1. Does the Good Samaritan law have legislation on AED use?

2. Who is covered or protected by the AED law?

3. Are there any training requirements of AED users? If so, describe these requirements.

Check-Call-Care Skill: CPR

CPR–ADULT

Step 1

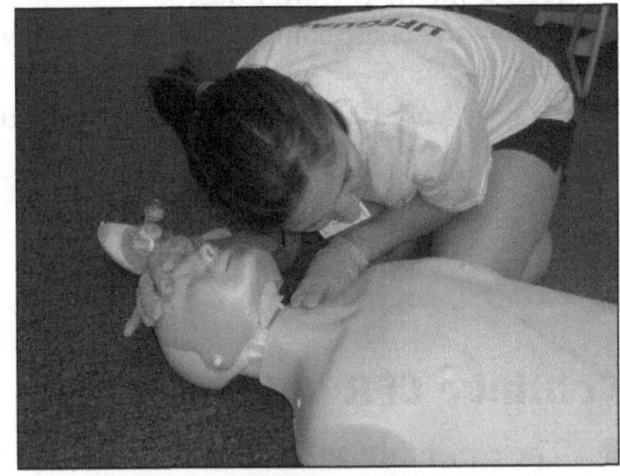
Figure 13.6

- Check level of consciousness (LOC).
- If the patient is unconscious, activate 9-1-1.
- Open the airway.
- Look, listen, and feel for breathing for no more than 10 seconds (Figure 13.6).

Step 2

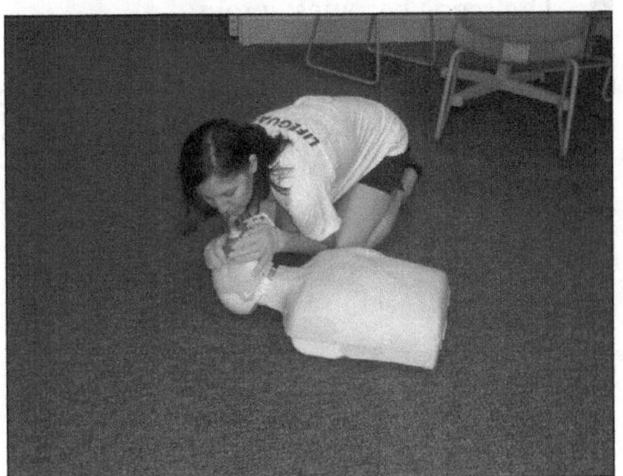
Figure 13.7

- If there is no breathing, give the patient two ventilations (Figure 13.7).
- If the ventilations go in, check for a carotid pulse.
- If the ventilations do not go in, retilt the head and give two additional ventilations.
- If the ventilations go in, check for a carotid pulse.

Expanded Chapter Content

Witnessed Sudden Collapse of an Adult

Please note that in a witnessed sudden collapse of an adult, quickly check for the presence of breathing and a pulse. If neither is present, begin chest compressions. The two initial ventilations are eliminated.

Step 3

- If there is no pulse, begin CPR.
- Place your dominant hand on the center of the patient's chest, across from the nipple line. Place your other hand over the dominant hand and interlock fingers.
- Keep elbows straight and give 30 chest compressions in about 18 seconds, depressing the chest at least 2 inches (Figure 13.8).
- Follow the chest compressions with two ventilations.
- Give at least 100 compressions per minute

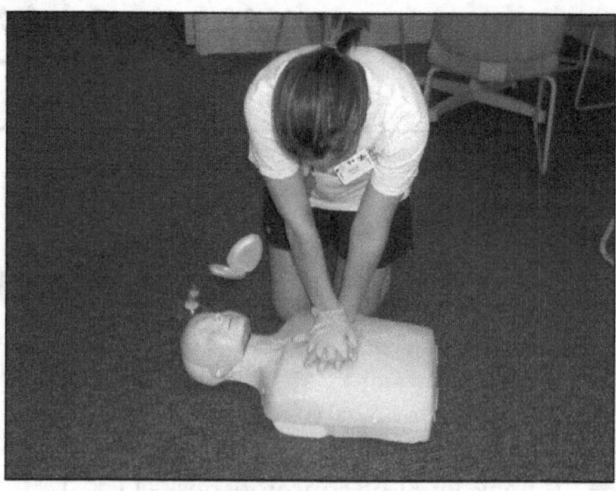

Figure 13.8

Continue CPR until:

- The patient shows signs of life
- Another trained rescuer takes over
- You are too exhausted to continue
- The scene becomes unsafe
- An AED becomes available
- You are presented with a valid DNR order
- More advanced medical personnel take over

CPR—CHILD

Step 1

- If the child is unconscious, activate 9-1-1.
- Open the airway.
- Look, listen, and feel for breathing for no more than 10 seconds (Figure 13.9).

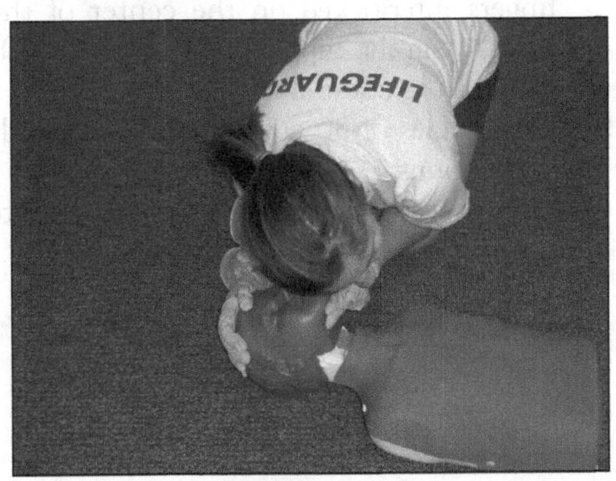

Figure 13.9

Step 2

- If the child is not breathing, give two ventilations (Figure 13.10).
- If the ventilations do not go in, retilt the head and give two additional ventilations.

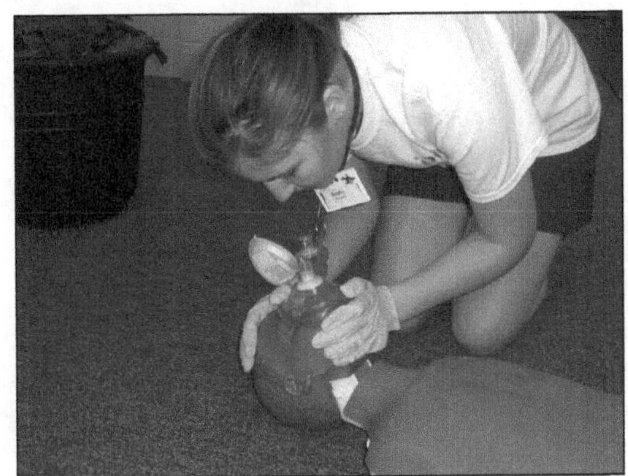

Figure 13.10

Step 3

- If the ventilations go in, check for a pulse for no more than 10 seconds (Figure 13.11).
- If there is no pulse, begin CPR.

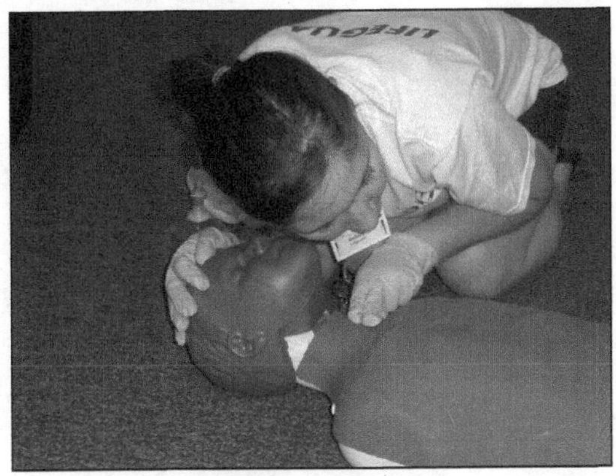

Figure 13.11

Step 4

- Find the correct hand position—two hands with fingers interlocked on the center of the chest, across from the nipple line (Figure 13.12).
- Depress the chest about 2 inches.
- Give cycles of 30 compressions followed by two ventilations.
- Give at least 100 compressions per minute.

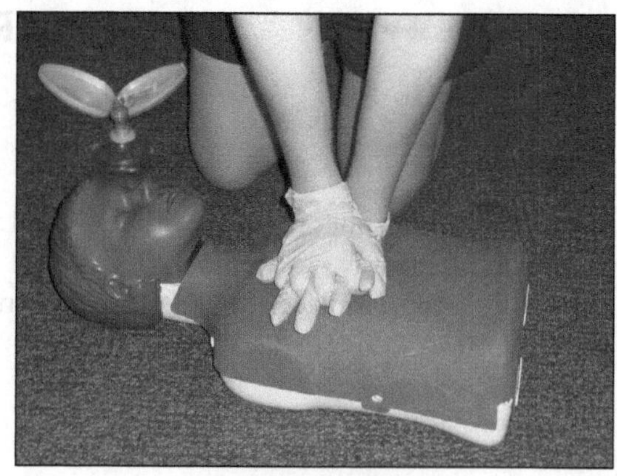

Figure 13.12

INFANT CPR

Step 1

- If the infant is unconscious; activate 9-1-1 (Figure 13.13).
- Open the airway.
- Look, listen, and feel for breathing for no more than 10 seconds (Figure 13.14).

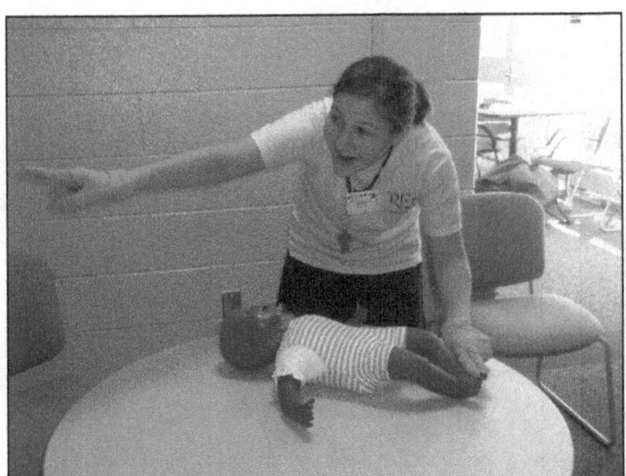

Figure 13.13

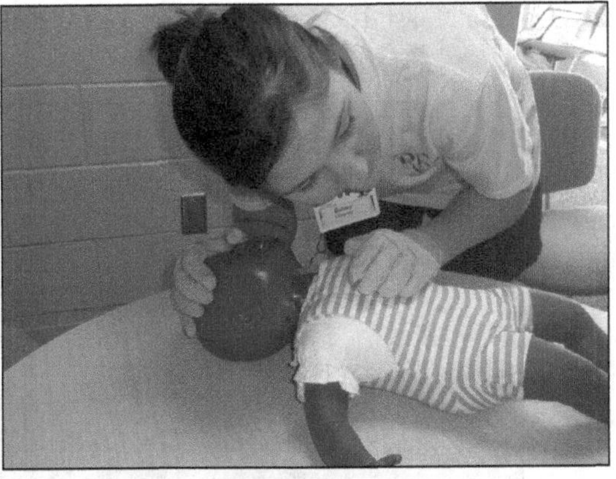

Figure 13.14

Step 2

- If the infant is not breathing, give two ventilations (Figure 13.15).
- If the ventilations do not go in, retilt the head and give two additional ventilations.

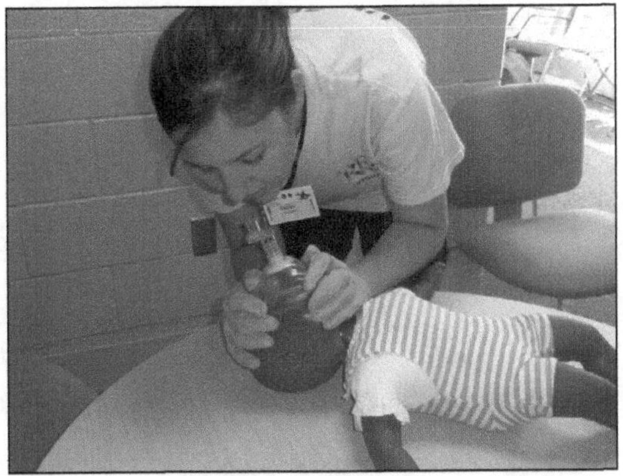

Figure 13.15

Step 3

- If the ventilations go in, check for a brachial pulse for no more than 10 seconds (Figure 13.16).
- If no pulse is felt, begin CPR.

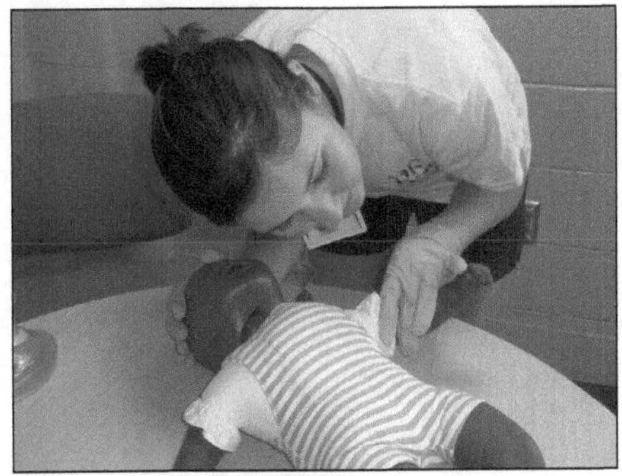

Figure 13.16

Step 4

- Position the infant on his/her back, on a firm, flat surface.
- Stand or kneel at the side of the infant's chest.
- Place one hand on the infant's forehead to keep the airway open, and two or three fingers of the other hand on the center of the infant's chest, slightly below the nipple line (Figures 13.17A and B).
- Keeping the fingers on the breastbone (sternum), depress the chest about 1½ inches.
- Give cycles of 30 compressions followed by two ventilations.
- Give at least 100 compressions per minute.

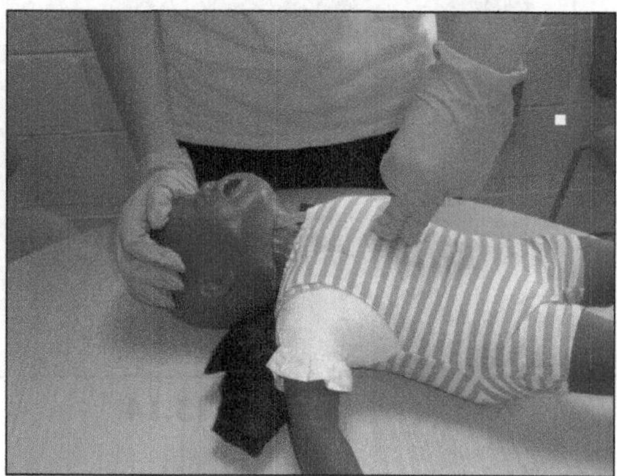

Figure 13.17A

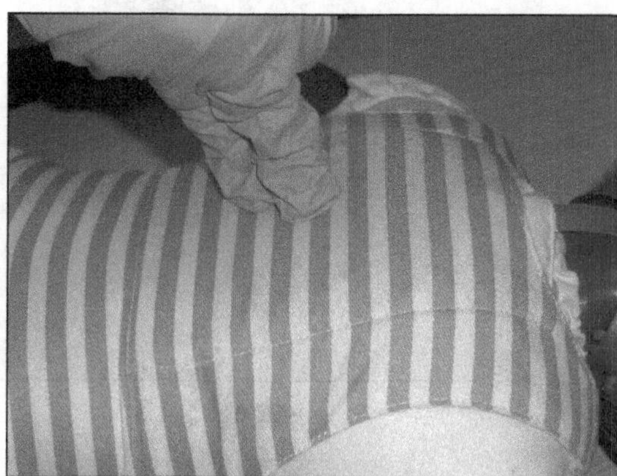

Figure 13.17B

TWO RESCUER CPR ADULT AND CHILD

One rescuer is performing CPR alone and a second rescuer arrives on the scene.

- The second rescuer states his/her name and level of training.
- The second rescuer asks if 9-1-1 has been activated. If not, the second rescuer activates 9-1-1 and brings an AED, if available. If 9-1-1 has been activated, the second rescuer should get an AED, if available.
- If an AED is not available, the second rescuer waits until the first rescuer moves to the head to give two ventilations, then places his/her hands on the center of the patient's chest and begins 30 chest compressions (15 compressions if the patient is a child or infant) (Figure 13.18).
- About every 2 minutes, the rescuer giving compressions calls for a change by substituting the word "change" for the number 30 (or 15).
- At the completion of 30 (or 15) compressions and 2 ventilations, the rescuers switch roles. The first rescuer moves from the head to the chest to deliver compressions while the second rescuer moves from the chest to the head to deliver ventilations.

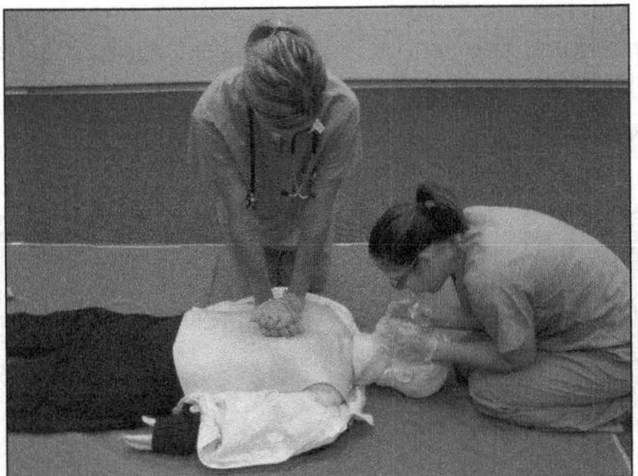

Figure 13.18

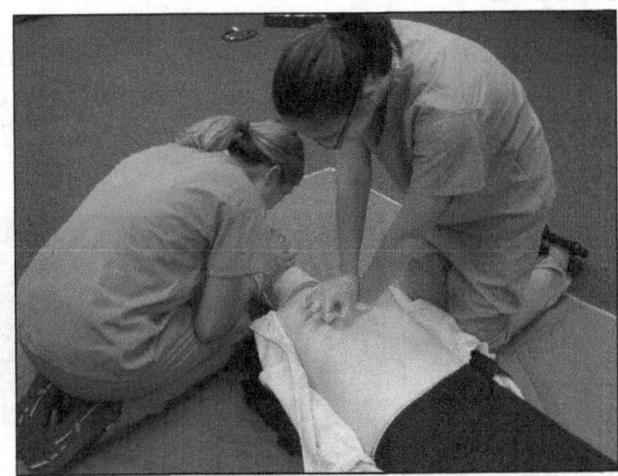

Figure 13.19

Two rescuers arrive at an emergency scene simultaneously.

- The first rescuer performs a primary (initial) assessment while the second rescuer activates 9-1-1 and gets an AED, if available.
- One rescuer assumes the role of ventilator while the other assumes the role of compressor.
- About every 2 minutes, the rescuer giving compressions calls for a change by substituting the word "change" for the number 30 (or 15).
- At the completion of 30 (or 15) compressions and 2 ventilations, the rescuers switch roles. The first rescuer moves from the head to the chest to deliver compressions while the second rescuer moves from the chest to the head to deliver ventilations.

TWO RESCUER CPR–INFANT

Step 1

- The first rescuer stands or kneels at the infant's feet and uses the "encircling hands" technique.
- Place your thumbs on the breastbone (sternum) just below the nipple line (Figure 13.20).
- Encircle the infant's chest with your fingers.
- Make sure that you do not compress or squeeze the ribs.

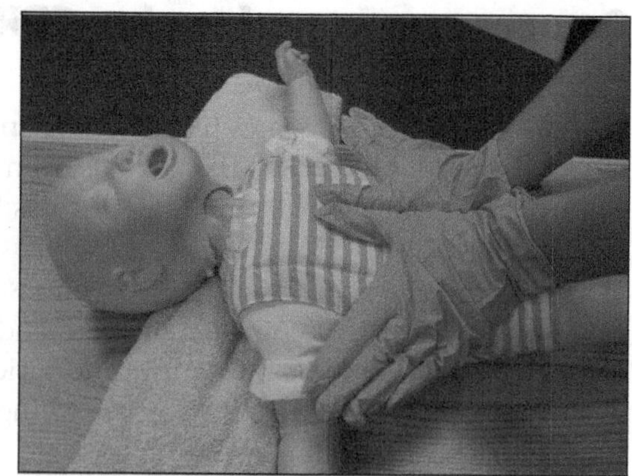

Figure 13.20

Step 2

- While the first rescuer is giving chest compressions, the second rescuer is positioned at the head of the infant to give two ventilations (Figures 13.21A and B).
- Continue cycles of 15 compressions and 2 ventilations.

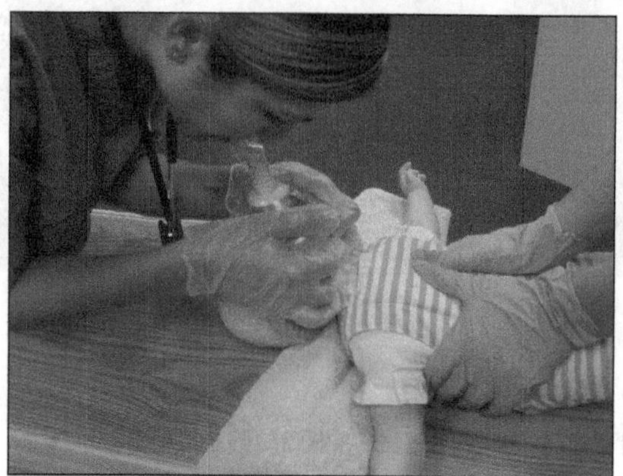

Figure 13.21A

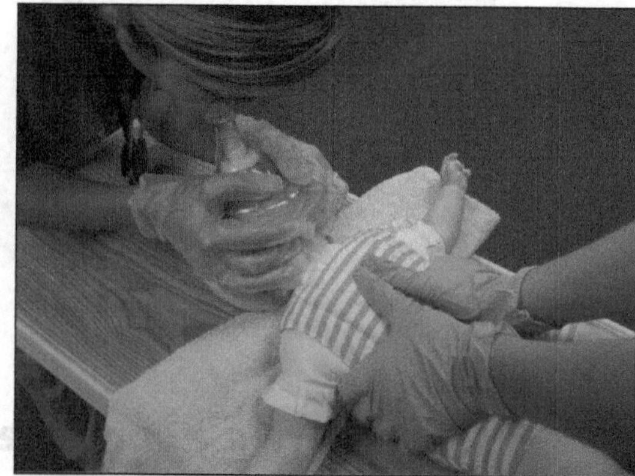

Figure 13.21B

Step 3

- The first rescuer (the compressor) calls for a change about every 2 minutes (Figure 13.22).
- At the end of 15 compressions, the second rescuer gives two ventilations and moves to the chest while the first rescuer moves from the chest to the head.

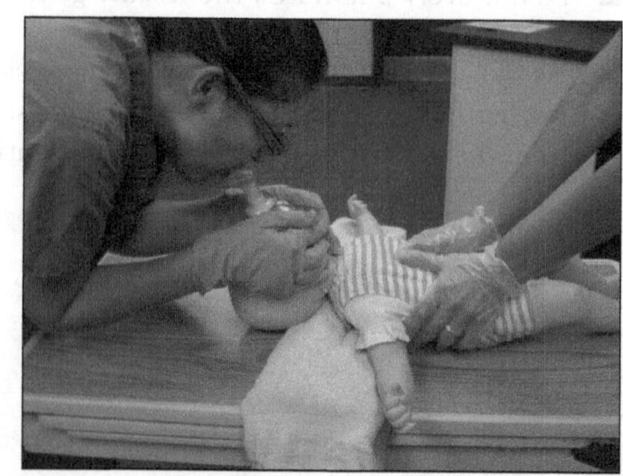

Figure 13.22

Expanded Chapter Content

Two Rescuer CPR – Child and Infant

The rationale for switching the ratio of compressions to ventilations from 30:2 to 15:2 in a child or infant during two rescuer CPR is because pediatric patients need additional oxygen at more frequent intervals.

USING AN AED – ADULT, CHILD, AND INFANT

Step 1

- Perform a primary (initial) assessment.
- If the patient is unconscious, activate 9-1-1.
- Turn on the AED (Figure 13.23).

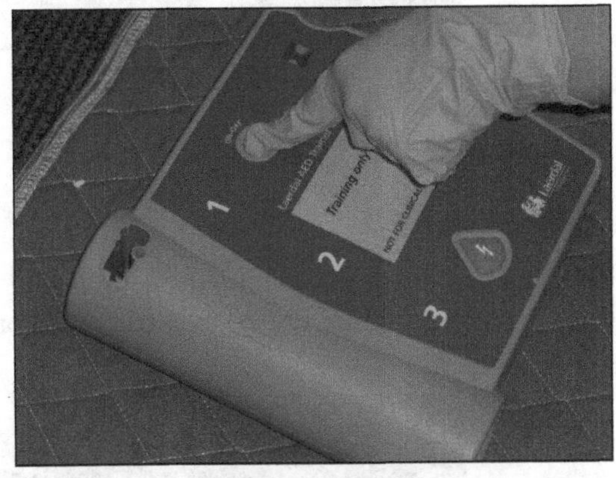

Figure 13.23

Step 2

- Wipe the patient's chest with a disposable towel (Figure 13.24).
- If there is a lot of chest hair, shave the areas where the pads are placed.

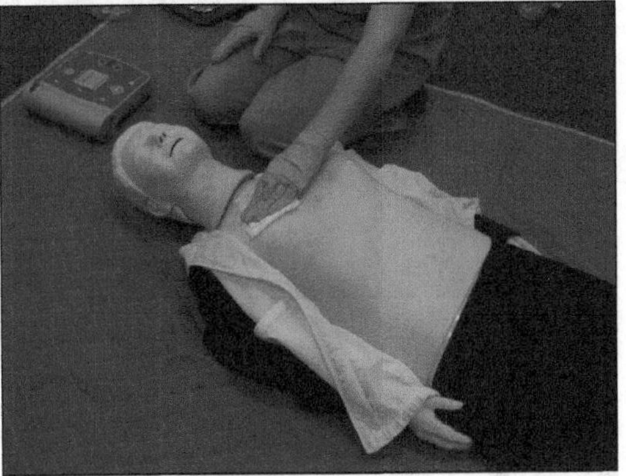

Figure 13.24

Step 3

- Apply pads to the chest; one pad on the patient's right upper shoulder and the second pad on the left side of the chest, just under the breast (Figure 13.25)
- **Child and infant:** Place one pad on the center of the chest and the second pad on the center of the back (Figures 13.26 and 13.27).

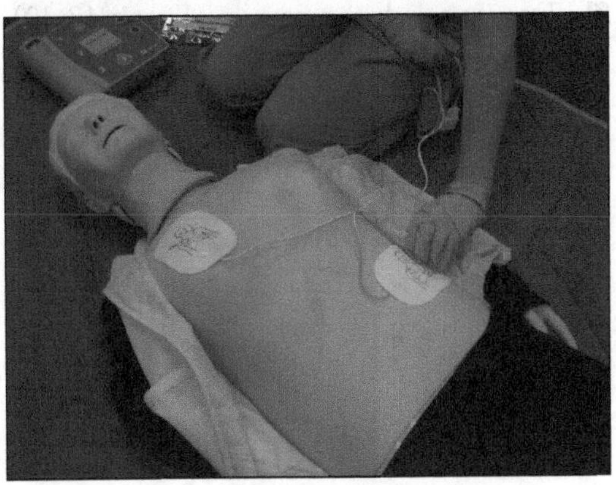

Figure 13.25

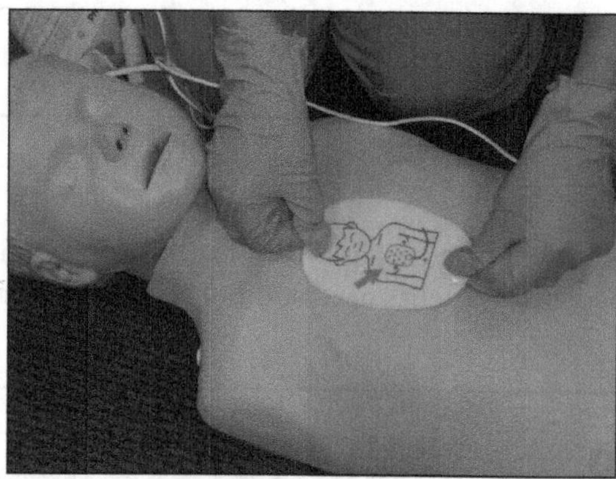

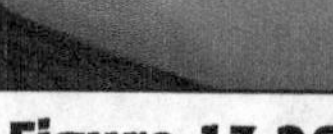

Figure 13.26

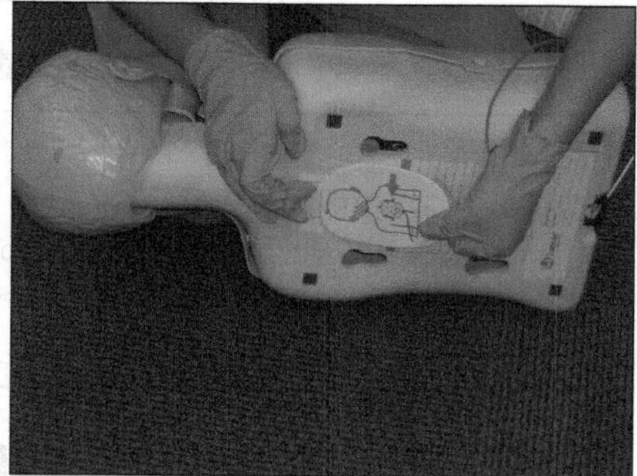

Figure 13.27

Step 4

- Plug in the connector (Figure 13.28).
- **Child and infant:** Use a pediatric AED or pediatric cables (Figure 13.29).

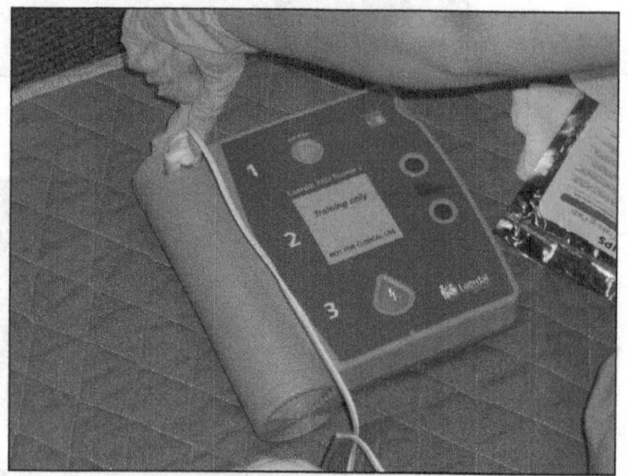

Figure 13.28

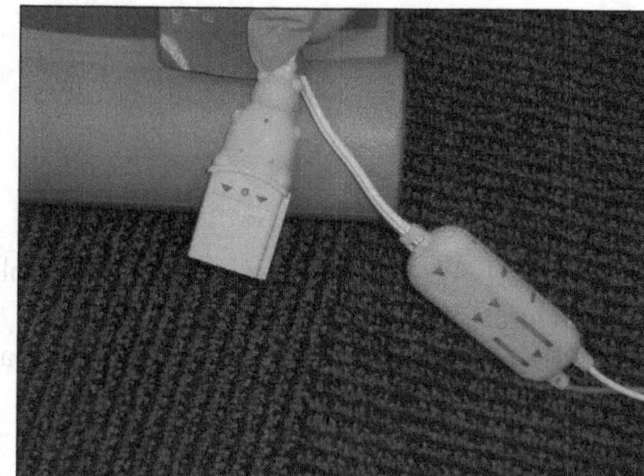

Figure 13.29

Step 5

- Allow the AED to analyze the heart rhythm.
- Do not touch the patient (Figure 13.30).

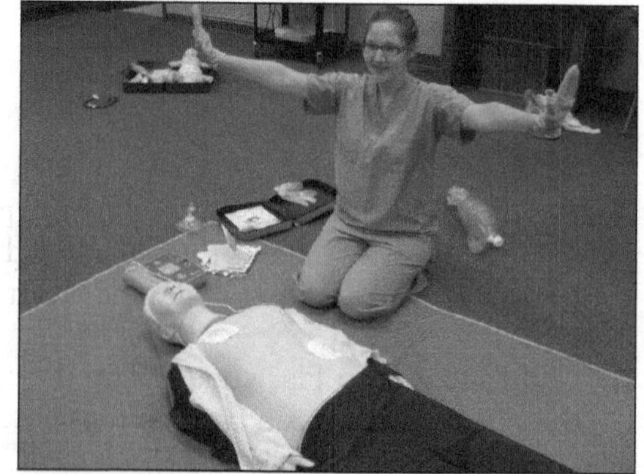

Figure 13.30

Step 6

- If a shock is advised, stand clear before pushing the shock button (Figure 13.31).

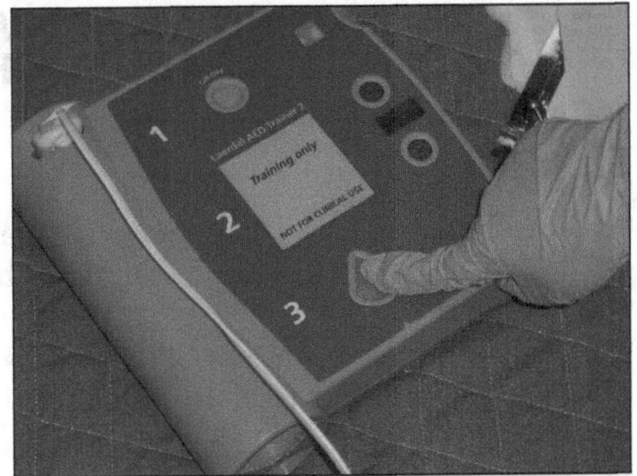

Figure 13.31

Step 7

- After delivering the shock, perform CPR if needed. Leave pads in place (Figure 13.32).
- At the end of 2 minutes, the AED will re-analyze the heart rhythm. Do not touch the patient.
    - If a shock is advised, follow steps 6 and 7.
    - If no shock is advised, perform 2 minutes of CPR if needed.

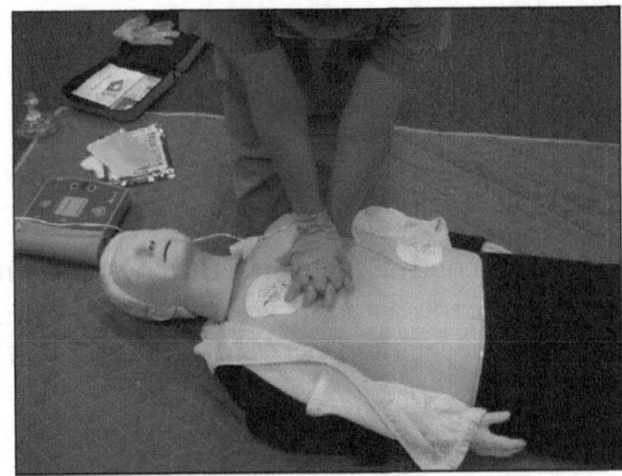

Figure 13.32

Expanded Chapter Content

CPR and the Use of the AED

If you are a lone rescuer with a victim who has no pulse and is not breathing, activate EMS and then apply the AED. If CPR is in progress and an AED becomes available, CPR should be continued until the AED is ready to analyze the heart rhythm. The first rescuer continues CPR while the second rescuer turns on the AED, wipes the patient's chest, applies the pads, and plugs in the connector. CPR should be stopped at this point since the machine is ready to analyze the heart rhythm.

USING AN AED WITH CPR IN PROGRESS–ADULT, CHILD, AND INFANT

Step 1

- The second rescuer identifies self by name and level of training and asks whether EMS has been activated.
- The first rescuer continues CPR. (CPR is continued until the AED is ready to analyze the heart rhythm.)
- The second rescuer turns on the AED (Figure 13.33).

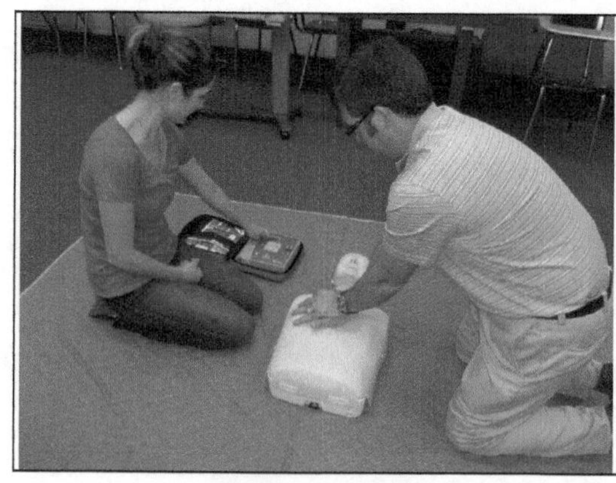

Figure 13.33

Step 2

- The second rescuer wipes the chest dry with a disposable towel and shaves the areas of the chest for pad placement, if necessary (Figure 13.34).

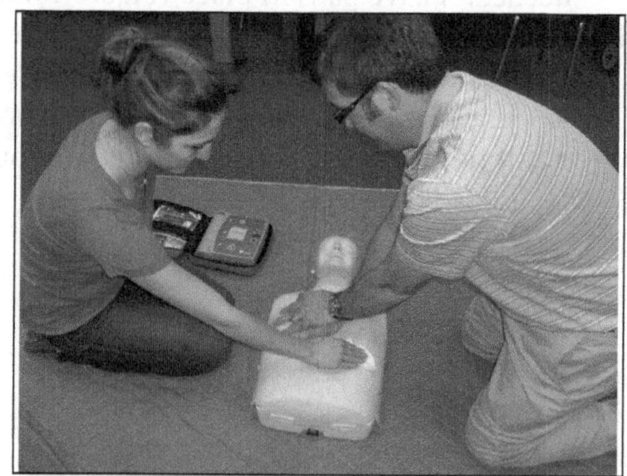

Figure 13.34

Step 3

- The second rescuer applies one pad on the patient's right upper shoulder area and the second pad on the left side of the chest, just under the breast (Figure 13.35).
- **Child and infant:** Apply pads as in Figures 13.26 and 13.27.

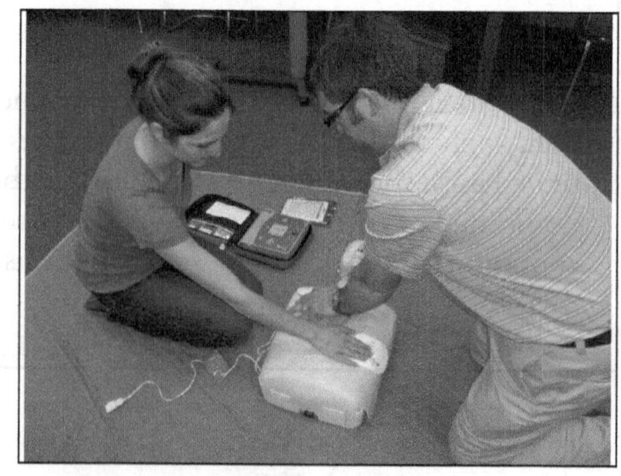

Figure 13.35

Step 4

- Plug in the connector (Figure 13.36).
- **Child and infant:** Use a pediatric AED or pediatric cables (Figure 13.29).

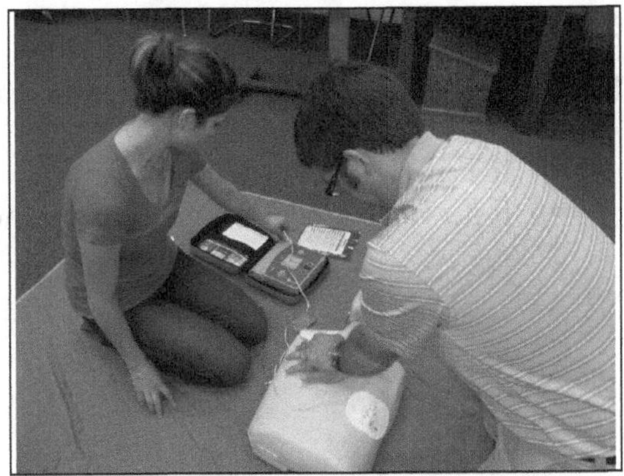

Figure 13.36

Step 5

- The second rescuer instructs the first rescuer to stop CPR.
- Allow the AED to analyze the heart rhythm.
- Make sure that no one is touching the patient (Figure 13.37).

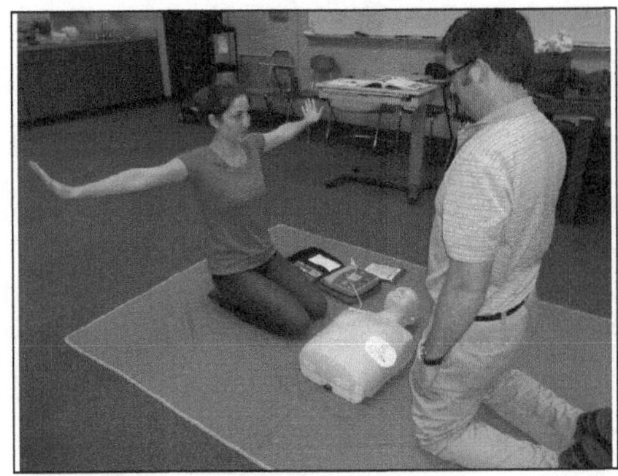

Figure 13.37

Step 6

- If a shock is advised, make sure no one is touching the patient, then depress the shock button (Figure 13.38).
- If no shock is advised, perform 2 minutes of CPR if necessary (Figure 13.39).

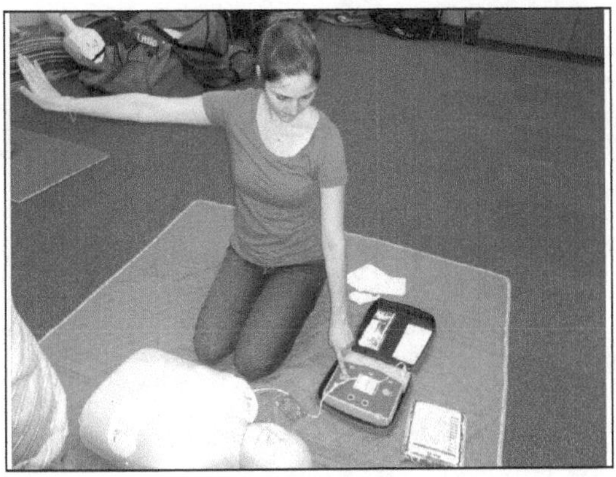

Figure 13.38

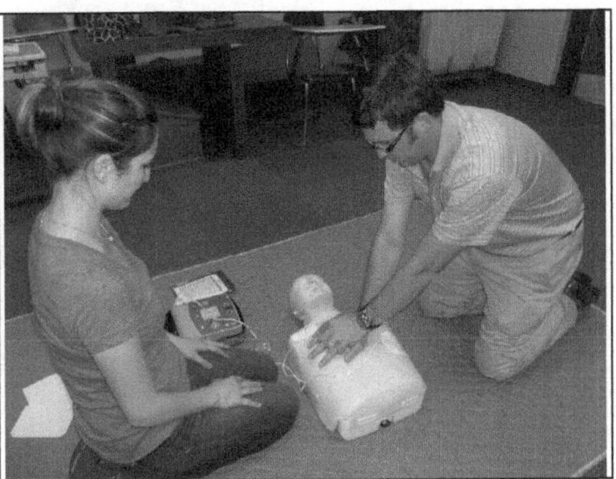

Figure 13.39

Step 7

- At the end of 2 minutes, the AED will reanalyze the heart rhythm. Stop CPR and make sure no one is touching the patient.
  - If a shock is advised, follow step 6.
  - If no shock is advised, perform 2 minutes of CPR if needed.

Unit 5

Medical Emergencies

14 Medical Emergencies

Expanded Chapter Content

- Seizures
- Stroke
- Diabetic Emergencies

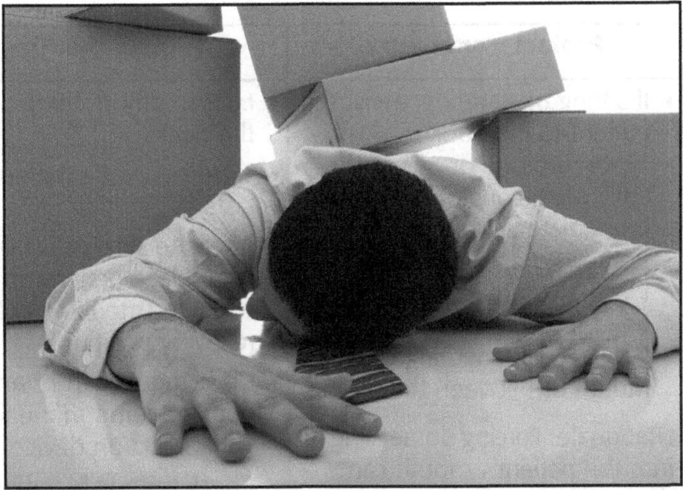

Chapter Significance

A medical emergency is a situation in which a patient experiences a sudden, unexpected illness. Medical emergencies can be caused by an *acute* (sudden) condition or develop as a consequence of a *chronic* (long term) condition. Although the causes are varied, many medical emergencies are associated with common chronic diseases, such as cardiovascular disease (primarily heart disease and stroke), high blood pressure (*hypertension*), epilepsy, and diabetes.

Even though the cause may be unknown and the presenting signs and symptoms similar, you can still provide appropriate care to the patient. Always follow the *standard of care* in treating conditions that you find. During the *primary assessment*, look for and treat *life-threatening conditions* and activate EMS immediately.

Remember: You do not have to "diagnose" the problem in order to treat the patient.

CHECK ▪ CALL ▪ CARE

911

Care of Seizure Patients

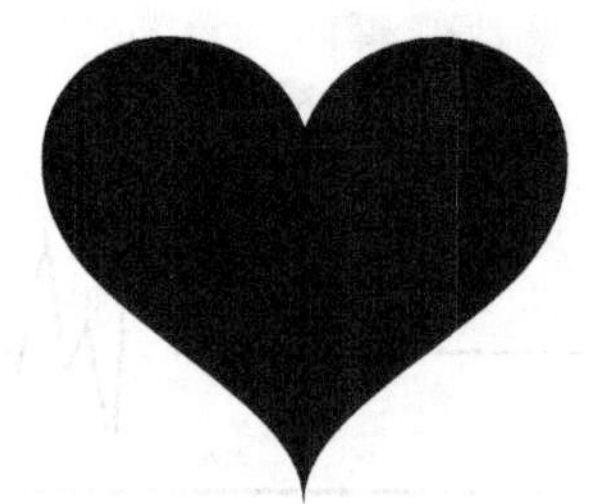

Although watching a person have a seizure can be frightening, remember that emergency care, regardless of the cause, is directed at three objectives:

- **Protect** the patient from injury
- **Protect** the patient's airway
- **Protect** the patient's privacy

Protect from Injury	Protect the Airway	Protect Privacy
• If sitting or standing, assist the patient to the floor. • Move furniture or any potentially dangerous objects in the immediate area. • Remove eyeglasses if worn. • Place a soft object under the head to cushion it. • Do **NOT** put anything into the mouth or between the teeth. (Rationale: Forcing something into the patient's mouth can damage the patient's jaw or teeth and injure the rescuer's fingers. Seizure patients rarely bite their tongues and tongues cannot be swallowed.) • Do **NOT** hold down or restrain the patient's body movements. Allow the seizure to run its course. Stay with the patient until fully conscious and aware of surroundings. • Perform a physical examination following the seizure to check for injuries (DOTS).	• Loosen any clothing around the neck. • Time how long the seizure lasts. • After the seizure activity is over, place patient on his or her side (modified H.A.IN.E.S. recovery position). • Clear the mouth of any secretions or vomit manually or with a suction device. • Check for any bleeding or injuries to the mouth. • Provide oxygen, if necessary, when available and trained to use.	• Instruct bystanders to move away from the area. • Place a blanket or any article of clothing over the patient in case of loss over bladder/bowel control.

The care is the same for a child experiencing a *febrile* seizure. Immediately following the seizure, cool the child by removing excess clothing and giving the child a sponge bath with lukewarm water. Acetominophen products can be administered to reduce a fever. Children under the age of 18 should not be given aspirin to reduce fevers because aspirin has been linked to the development of Reye's syndrome, a potentially fatal disease involving the internal organs and brain.

Stroke

A call was received by the local EMS agency from a 60-year-old female who reported a sudden onset of numbness and tingling to the left side of her face and arm. She stated that the symptoms disappeared as quickly as they started, lasting only a matter of seconds. She reported no confusion nor the loss of strength or movement in her arm. Several weeks after this episode, findings from a brain scan confirmed that this woman had a stroke.

Public Health Burden

In the United States, a stroke occurs every 40 seconds. According to the American Heart Association, stroke is the fourth leading cause of death in the United States, killing more than 140,000 individuals annually. It is a leading cause of chronic disability, afflicting approximately 795,000 Americans each year. The American Heart Association estimates that the projected costs for stroke patients in 2009 will exceed $68 billion. About 75% of all strokes occur in people over the age of 65. The risk of having a stroke more than doubles each decade after the age of 55. High blood pressure (*hypertension*) is the most important risk factor for the development of a stroke.

What Is a Stroke?

Medically referred to as a ***cerebrovascular accident* (CVA),** a stroke is a disturbance in the brain's blood supply, which occurs when a blood vessel becomes blocked or when a blood vessel bursts. Permanent brain damage may result if treatment is delayed more than a few hours.

Types of Strokes

Ischemic stroke

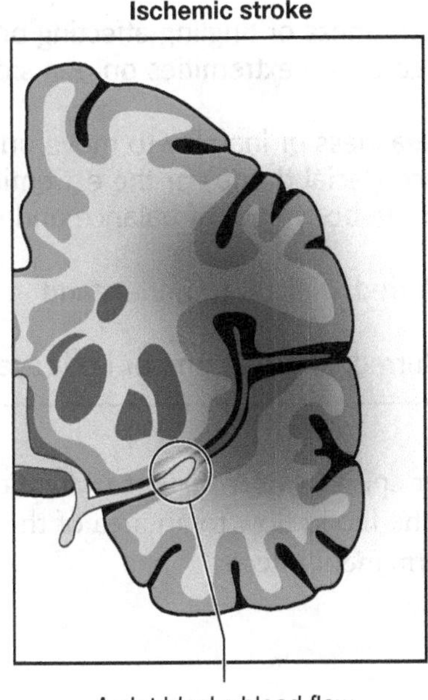

A clot blocks blood flow to an area of the brain

Hemorrhagic stroke

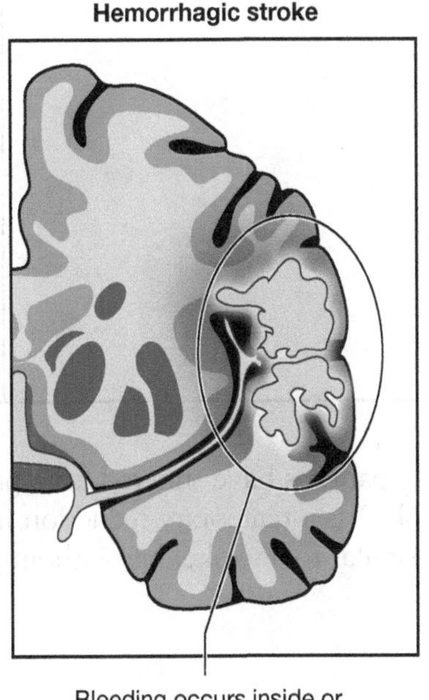

Bleeding occurs inside or around brain tissue

There are two types of stroke: ***ischemic stroke*** and ***hemorrhagic stroke.***

An ischemic stroke is more common in people 65 years of age and older, accounting for approximately 85% of all strokes. This type of stroke occurs when blood flow to the brain is blocked or obstructed. The blockage may come from a blood clot (***thrombus*** or ***embolus***) or from fatty plaque deposits associated with atherosclerosis. When the blood flow through a major artery is blocked, areas of the brain will receive less oxygenated blood, altering brain function and, in some cases, causing permanent brain damage.

A hemorrhagic stroke occurs when a blood vessel in the brain ruptures or leaks, causing bleeding into the brain. Hemorrhagic strokes are less common but more deadly than ischemic strokes, contributing to more than 30% of all stroke deaths. Poorly controlled hypertension and ruptured cerebral aneurysms are among the causes of hemorrhagic strokes. An ***aneurysm*** refers to a weakening of the muscular wall of an artery, causing it to bulge and eventually rupture.

Check the Patient: Warning Signs and Symptoms of a Stroke

It is important to recognize the major signs and symptoms of a stroke and determine when they started. Time is critical with a stroke patient to preserve brain function. Prompt diagnosis and medical treatment can save a patient's life and limit the number of patients who are faced with long-term disabilities. The warning signs and symptoms of a stroke have a sudden onset and typically affect the following body functions.

Area of Body Function	Altered Behavior
• Mental Status	Dizziness, drowsiness, confusion, mood change, loss of consciousness, severe headache
• Sensation	Numbness or tingling affecting one side of the face or the extremities on one side of the body
• Movement	Weakness or inability to move one side of the face (facial droop) or the extremities on one side of the body; loss of balance and coordination
• Speech	Slurred, difficult to understand
• Vision	Blurred, affecting one or both eyes

Frequently, stroke patients have suffered from prior episodes of ***transient ischemic attacks (TIAs)***. A TIA, or "mini-stroke," is a temporary reduction in the blood flow to an area of the brain that causes signs and symptoms similar to a stroke, but without permanent effects.

If you think that someone might be having a stroke, act quickly and use this simple stroke assessment tool, based on the **Cincinnati Prehospital Stroke Scale**. This scale was developed in 1997 for EMS personnel.

ACT F.A.S.T.		
	Instructions to Patient	**Findings**
Face	Ask the patient to smile.	**Normal:** both sides of face move equally (Figure 14.1) **Abnormal:** one side of the face does not move; facial droop (see Figure 14.2)
Arms	Ask the patient to close his or her eyes and raise both arms out in front of the body.	**Normal:** both arms move equally or not at all (see Figure 14.3) **Abnormal:** one arm drops or shifts downward (see Figure 14.4)
Speech	Ask the patient to repeat a simple sentence: "A rolling stone gathers no moss."	**Normal:** uses correct words with no slurring **Abnormal:** speech is slurred or garbled; uses inappropriate word; lacks the ability to speak (aphasic).
Time	Time is critical!! Call 9-1-1 if someone shows any of these signs.	
Source: Adapted from National Stroke Association: What is Stroke		

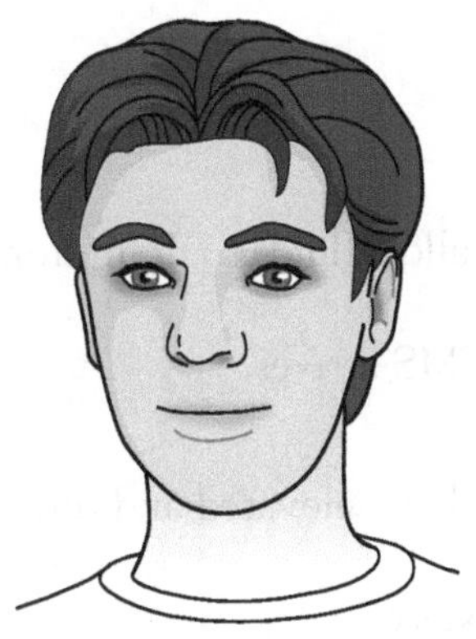

Figure 14.1
Facial Symmetry

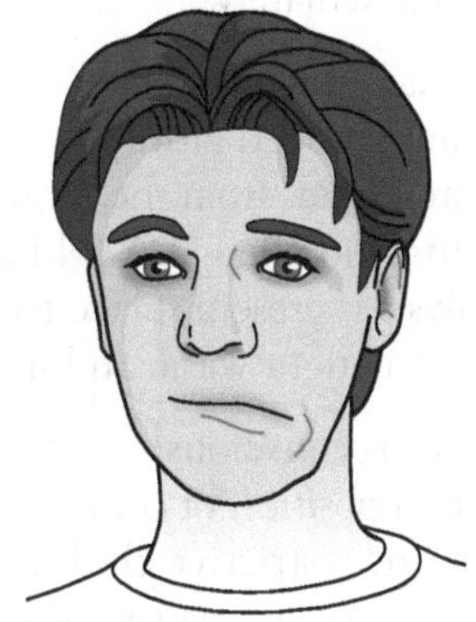

Figure 14.2
Facial Droop

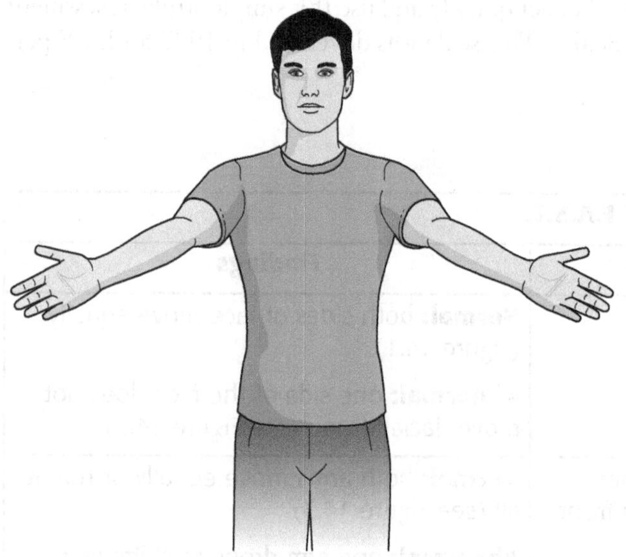

Figure 14.3
Arm Symmetry

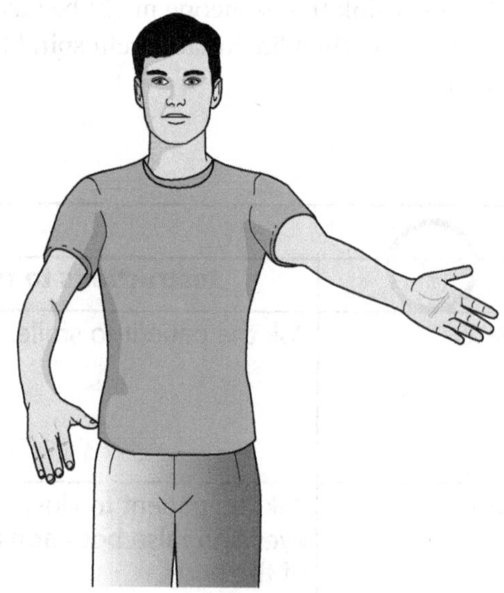

Figure 14.4
Arm Asymmetry

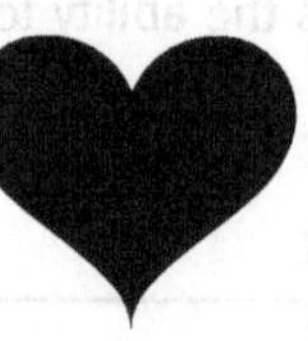

Emergency Care for a Stroke Patient

The key elements to successful stroke management are the rapid identification of the stroke and rapid transport to a hospital or stroke center. Prompt medical care can limit permanent brain damage, but some treatments are time sensitive. One such treatment is the intravenous use of recombinant tissue plasminogen activator (t-PA), a powerful drug that quickly dissolves the blood clot causing an ischemic stroke. However, the currently approved time limit for administration of this drug to stroke patients is 3 hours from the time of symptom onset.

Based upon your assessment, if a stroke is suspected, follow these steps for care:

1. Call 9-1-1 immediately.
2. If the patient is **unconscious:**
   - Maintain an open airway
   - Clear any fluids from the mouth.
   - Place in a modified H.A.IN.E.S. recovery position to allow fluids to drain from the mouth.
   - If paralysis is present, place the paralyzed side down.
   - Keep the patient warm and monitor the ABCs until EMS arrives.
3. If the patient is **conscious:**
   - Place in a position of comfort, lying on the back with head elevated and turned to the side.
   - Loosen any restrictive clothing around the neck.
   - Be calm and offer reassurance to decrease fear and anxiety.
   - Use nonverbal ways to communicate (hand squeezing, eye blinking) and brief questions that require only "yes" or "no" responses.
   - Do not give anything to eat or drink.

Diabetic Emergencies: The High and the Low

What Is Diabetes?

Diabetes mellitus is a group of metabolic conditions characterized by high levels of blood glucose (***hyperglycemia***), caused by defects in insulin production, insulin utilization, or both. The hormone insulin, produced by the pancreas, is needed by certain cells of the body to use glucose. In 2010, approximately 27% of the population in the United States aged 65 and older had diabetes. About 1 in 400 children and adolescents have diabetes. In the United States, diabetes is the leading cause of kidney failure, lower-limb amputations, and new cases of blindness among adults. Diabetes is the major cause of heart disease and stroke and the seventh leading cause of death in the United States.

Here is an easy way to understand what happens in diabetes.

Think of a cell as a door that is locked. Insulin can be viewed as the key which unlocks the door (cell membrane), allowing glucose to enter the cell for energy production. Some individuals with diabetes lack enough "keys" (insulin) to unlock the doors (cell membranes); without glucose, a cell cannot carry out its functions and will die. Other individuals with diabetes develop a resistance to insulin; their body is making enough insulin (keys) but the keys don't fit the lock; the door doesn't open and glucose cannot get in, causing cell death. When either or both of these conditions occur, the glucose or sugar levels rise in the blood causing damage to organs such as the heart (heart attack), eyes (*retinopathy* causing blindness), kidneys (kidney failure leading to *dialysis*), nervous system (*neuropathy* causing numbness and tingling of the hands and feet), and erectile dysfunction in men

Types of Diabetes

There are two major types of diabetes: ***type 1*** and ***type 2***. Type 1 diabetes (formerly called insulin-dependent diabetes mellitus [IDDM] or juvenile-onset diabetes) develops when the body's immune system fails, attacking and destroying the pancreatic cells that produce insulin. Due to the destruction, the pancreas produces little or no insulin. Therefore, people with type 1 diabetes rely on an outside source of insulin, primarily in the form of injections, in order to survive.

Type 2 diabetes (formerly called non-insulin-dependent diabetes mellitus [NIDDM] or adult-onset diabetes) is associated with advancing age and accounts for more than 90% of all diabetes cases. Type 2 diabetes can be prevented, since the increase in the number of cases is linked closely to the obesity epidemic in the United States. Type 2 diabetes usually begins as insulin resistance, a problem with insulin use, but eventually develops into a reduction in insulin production. The increase in obesity among adolescents and young adults is predisposing them to the development of type 2 diabetes, usually seen in middle age.

Gestational diabetes, a form of diabetes that can develop in pregnant women, often goes away after the birth of the baby. All pregnant women are tested for gestational diabetes because it can lead to large birth weight infants (>10 pounds).

Managing Diabetic Emergencies

People who have diabetes routinely experience problems with glucose control. Because the body's demand for insulin can vary from moment to moment—depending upon the person's food intake, amount of physical activity, stress, or the presence of an infection—the blood sugar levels can fluctuate. When the insulin level is too high, blood sugar levels can drop dangerously low, called **hypoglycemia**. When the insulin level is too low, blood sugar levels can climb dangerously high, called **hyperglycemia**.

Diabetes is becoming more common in the United States, affecting more than 23 million people of all ages. It is important that emergency medical responders, as well as the general public, be able to recognize the signs and symptoms of hypoglycemia and hyperglycemia and how to respond correctly.

SIGNS AND SYMPTOMS OF DIABETIC EMERGENCIES	
Hypoglycemia	**Hyperglycemia**
• Low blood sugar • Insulin shock	• High blood sugar • Diabetic coma, diabetic ketoacidosis
• *Skin:* pale, sweating • *Nervous system changes:* headache, drowsiness, confusion, lightheaded, weak, tremors, seizures • *Mood changes:* irritability, shaky, or anxious • Blurred vision *often mistaken for being drunk *tends to have a rapid onset	• *Skin:* dry, flushed • Look for "*3 POLYs*": Polyuria (frequent urination) Polydipsia (excessive thirst) Polyphagia (extreme hunger) • *Nervous system changes:* headache, drowsiness, confusion, loss of consciousness, seizures • *Breathing:* rapid and deep; fruity smelling breath • Nausea and vomiting *develops slowly

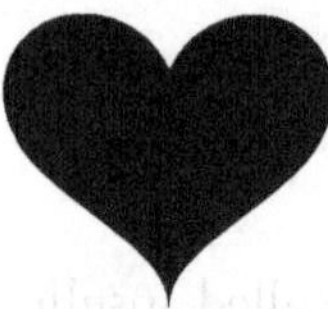

Care for Diabetic Emergencies

Although they are different conditions, many of the signs and symptoms of hypoglycemia and hyperglycemia are the same. Therefore, based upon your assessment, you may not know what the problem is. However, it will be helpful to **REMEMBER** two things:

- You do not need to diagnose the problem in order to care for the patient.
- The brain requires a constant supply of glucose. When in doubt, treat the patient for a low blood sugar and GIVE GLUCOSE!

Treatment of hypoglycemia: Give glucose. The goal is to provide 15 grams of carbohydrate (as a rapidly dissolving food product) to raise the blood sugar level quickly (in about 15 minutes). This is referred to as the "rule of 15."

1. If the patient is **alert and able to swallow:**
   - Give a simple sugar that is rapidly absorbed into the body (also known as a quick-fix food): ½ c. fruit juice, ½ can regular soft drink, 1 c. milk, 5-6 pieces of hard candy, 1 T. honey, 3-4 glucose tablets, 1 serving of glucose gel or paste, or 2 T sugar dissolved in several ounces of water.
   - If signs and symptoms are still present after 15 minutes, give more sugar. If the condition improves, follow the initial treatment with a protein/complex carbohydrate meal or snack (cheese, cottage cheese, meat sandwich, peanut butter and crackers).
   - If no improvement or the condition worsens, call 9-1-1.
2. If the patient is **unable to swallow or is unresponsive:**
   - Do **NOT** give anything to eat or drink.
   - Call 9-1-1 immediately.
   - Place in a modified H.A.IN.E.S. recovery position and monitor the ABCs.

Sources

American Diabetes Association www.diabetes.org/diabetes-basics/diabetes-statistics/

American Heart Association. Heart Disease and Stroke Statistics – 2009 Update. Dallas, Tex., 2009. www.americanheart.org

American Heart Association and the American National Red Cross (2010). Part 17: First aid: 2010 American Heart Association and American Red Cross Guidelines for First Aid. *Circulation* 122:S934-S946. http://circ.ahajournals.org/content/122/18_suppl_3/S394

American Red Cross. *Emergency Medical Response*. Boston: StayWell. 2011.

American Stroke Association: A Division of American Heart Association. www.strokeassociation.org

Centers for Disease Control and Prevention: Division for Heart Disease and Stroke Prevention, National Center for Chronic Disease and Prevention. www.cdc.gov

Centers for Disease Control and Prevention. National diabetes fact sheet: general information and national estimates on diabetes in the United States, 2007. Atlanta, GA: U.S. Department of Health and Human Services, Centers for Disease Control and Prevention, 2008.

Kothari RU, Pancioli A, Liu T, Broderick J. Cincinnati Prehospital Stroke Scale: reproducibility and validity. *Ann Emerg Med*. 1999 Apr: 33, 4: 373-378.

National Diabetes Information Clearinghouse (NDIC) https://diabetes.niddk.nih.gov/dm/pubs/statistics/

National Institute of Neurological Disorders and Stroke. Seizures and epilepsy: hope through research, NINDS. Publication date May 2004. www.ninds.nih.gov

National Stroke Association www.stroke.org

Name: ______________________ Date: __________

Learning Activities

I. Multiple Choice

1. When someone is unsure whether a diabetic patient is experiencing hyperglycemia or hypoglycemia, the correct action would be to
   a. Contact the family to discuss the situation
   b. Administer insulin, if you are authorized
   c. Call the person's physician
   d. Give some form of glucose

2. To prevent injury in a person having a seizure, the emergency medical responder should
   a. Put an object in the mouth, between the teeth
   b. Place something soft and thick under the head
   c. Instruct bystanders to hold down the patient's arms and legs
   d. Place the patient in a sitting position

3. Which of the following positions would be best to place an unresponsive stroke patient?
   a. Sitting straight up
   b. Lying on one side
   c. Lying on the stomach
   d. Lying flat with legs raised

4. Following a seizure, the patient is typically
   a. Sleepy
   b. Comatose
   c. Hyperexcitable
   d. Agitated

5. Summoning more advanced medical personnel during or after a seizure is necessary if
   a. The seizure takes place in water
   b. The person is tired post-seizure
   c. The person has epilepsy
   d. The seizure is heat-induced

6. The recovery phase of the seizure is called the
   a. Aura phase
   b. Conic phase
   c. Clonic phase
   d. Post-ictal phase

7. A seizure that occurs following a fever in an infant or child is referred to as a(n)
   a. Febrile seizure
   b. Complex partial seizure
   c. Simple partial seizure
   d. Absence seizure

8. The blood sugar levels in a patient with type 1 diabetes can be controlled by
   a. Diet alone
   b. Diet and oral medications
   c. Insulin injections
   d. Oral medications

9. If you suspect that a patient has low blood sugar, which of the following actions would be most appropriate to take initially?
   a. Call 9-1-1.
   b. Give the patient 6 ounces of juice or pop to drink.
   c. Give the patient a meat sandwich to eat.
   d. Give the patient a peanut butter and jelly sandwich to eat.

10. A patient who has problems with blood sugar levels has a problem with which body system?
   a. Circulatory
   b. Digestive
   c. Endocrine
   d. Urinary

11. You are assessing a patient who has kidney failure and is receiving hemodialysis three times per week. The patient has been ill and has gone without hemodialysis for 5 days. What sign would you expect to see in your assessment of the patient?
   a. Generalized edema
   b. Hypotension
   c. Tachycardia
   d. Flushed, dry skin

12. You arrive at the scene of an emergency and find that the patient is in status epilepticus. Your first action would be to
   a. Administer emergency oxygen
   b. Suction the patient's mouth
   c. Place the patient in a modified H.A.IN.E.S. recovery position
   d. Summon more advanced medical personnel

13. Which of the following actions would be most appropriate for an emergency medical responder to do when assessing and providing care to a patient who has had a stroke?
   a. Use a finger sweep on a conscious patient who vomited during the stroke.
   b. If fluid or vomit is in an unresponsive stroke patient's mouth, position him or her on one side to allow fluids to drain out of the mouth.
   c. Try to get the patient to speak as much as possible.
   d. If the patient is conscious, place in a supine position.

14. You are providing care to a patient having a seizure. Which of the following actions would be a priority?
   a. Offering comfort and reassurance
   b. Maintaining an open airway
   c. Putting an object in the mouth to prevent the patient from biting the tongue
   d. Positioning the patient in the supine position

15. A stroke can best be defined as
    a. A temporary episode due to reduced blood flow to the brain
    b. A condition having a sudden onset and rapid disappearance of symptoms
    c. A disruption of blood flow to a part of the brain, which may cause permanent damage to brain tissue
    d. A condition that causes irreversible brain damage each time

16. You are assessing an older adult for signs and symptoms of a stroke using the FAST mnemonic. What does the "T" stand for?
    a. The patient is unable to keep both arms raised.
    b. The patient is able to repeat words clearly and correctly.
    c. Drooling was observed from the left side of the patient's mouth.
    d. The onset of the symptoms was 1 hour ago.

II. Short Answer

1. An unusual sensation or feeling that frequently precedes generalized seizures is called an ______________.

2. The hormone that allows certain cells of the body to use glucose (sugar) is ____________________.

3. The acronym CVA stands for____________________ ____________________ ____________________.

4. A thrombus is a ____.

5. A weakened area of an artery in the brain that can balloon out and rupture, causing a stroke, is called an ____________________.

6. Name the two most common types of strokes.

   1.

   2.

7. An ounce of prevention is worth a pound of cure. Describe four lifestyle changes you can make to reduce the risk of stroke.

   1.

   2.

   3.

   4.

8. Describe the meaning of each letter in the FAST mnemonic.

   F = ______________________________

   A = ______________________________

   S = ______________________________

   T = ______________________________

9. Name and describe the two types of dialysis used to filter waste products from the patient's bloodstream.

   1.

   2.

III. True or False

_______ 1. When caring for a seizure patient, place something between the patient's teeth to prevent damage to the tongue.

_______ 2. In order to provide appropriate care for a person experiencing a medical emergency, it is not necessary to diagnose the specific illness.

_______ 3. A person who feels lightheaded and about to faint should lie down with the legs elevated.

_______ 4. It is necessary to call 9-1-1 for anyone having a seizure.

_______ 5. An ammonia inhalant can be used to arouse a person who has fainted.

_______ 6. The mnemonic FAST is used to assess seizure patients.

_______ 7. The most common cause of strokes is due to the rupture or leaking of blood vessels within the brain.

_______ 8. A person having a seizure might swallow his or her tongue.

_______ 9. During a seizure, stiffening of the arms and legs is referred to as tonic muscle activity.

IV. Scenarios

Scenario 1
You are an instructor in a first aid class. During the middle of a lesson, you suddenly hear a student sitting in the front row cry out loud and then start to jerk violently. (Questions 1–4 refer to Scenario 1.)

1. Identify two priorities of first aid management for this patient.

   1.

   2.

2. Based upon the information provided, would you call 9-1-1?
   Provide a rationale for your answer.

3. What specific actions will you take in meeting the priorities that you identified in question 1?

4. After the seizure has stopped, the best position to place the student would be
   a. Lying on her side
   b. Lying face down with head turned to the side
   c. Lying on her back with legs raised
   d. Lying in the modified H.A.IN.E.S. position

Scenario 2

Matt, 24 years of age and a diabetic since the age of 8, is driving home from work with several co-workers. He just finished a 12-hour day on a landscaping project in 85° weather. He is exhausted and sweating profusely. When he begins to have problems driving the car, his co-workers ask that he pull over to the side of the road. Matt complains that is vision is blurry and he feels weak and shaky. (Questions 1–4 refer to Scenario 2.)

1. Identify the problem(s) Matt is most likely experiencing?

2. List the signs and symptoms **in the scenario** that led you to arrive at the conclusions cited in question 1.

3. What questions would you ask Matt to help you better decide what is wrong?

4. What care should be provided to Matt to treat the problems identified in question 1?

Scenario 3
A dangerous ritual is about to begin – 21 drinks for the 21st birthday. A group of close friends has gathered for a special party for the "birthday boy." Everyone knows it is a dangerous game, but this is the so-called "right of passage" into adulthood. The activities begin, and the guest of honor is soon "chugging beers" and chasing them with shots of liquor. Two hours after the drinking began, you arrive at the party. The "birthday boy" is vomiting violently in the bathroom. Suddenly, he slumps to the floor and begins having violent convulsions. (Questions 1–3 relate to Scenario 3.)

1. What is wrong with this patient?

2. What are your two major priorities in providing care to this patient?

3. What care would you provide to this patient? Be specific.

Scenario 4
An elderly woman loses her balance and collapses to the floor in a supermarket. You hear the commotion in the next aisle and rush over. You find that the woman is lethargic and difficult to arouse. Her eyes are open and the left side of her face is drooping. She is making mumbling sounds but you cannot decipher her words. She has also vomited. (Questions 1–3 refer to Scenario 4.)

1. What medical emergency do you think this woman is having?

2. Would you activate EMS for this patient? Provide a rationale for your answer.

3. What specific care would you provide for this patient?

15 Poisoning

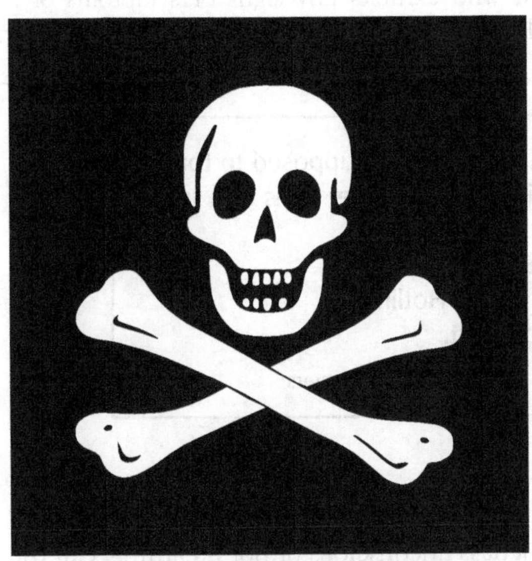

Chapter Significance

Every day in the United States, about 87 people die from unintentional poisoning and 2,277 people are treated in emergency departments. In 2010, poison control centers reported receiving 2.4 million calls related to poison exposure. Nearly 4.6 million people were seen in emergency departments nationwide in 2009 for drug-related problems; half were due to adverse effects from drugs and the other half were due to drug abuse. Approximately 32% of drug-abuse emergency department visits also involved the use of alcohol. Unintentional poisoning fatalities have steadily risen since 1992, ranking second only to motor vehicle accidents as a leading cause of accidental death in the United States. Among people between the ages of 25 and 64, unintentional poisonings caused more deaths than motor vehicle crashes.

Although some poisonings are intentional, caused by a deliberate attempt to harm oneself or another person, most poison exposures are unintentional and occur in the home. Most people automatically think of children when asked about poisoning problems. Emergency department

visits related to poisonings occur most frequently in children < 6 years of age. Adults tend to suffer more serious injuries and deaths from poisonings than children. 80% of poisoning deaths occur between the ages of 20 and 54 (CDC).

This chapter discusses various types of poisoning emergencies. Although most cases of poisoning involve substances that are swallowed, poisons can also be inhaled, absorbed, or injected. Knowing how to recognize and care for patients with a suspected poisoning, as well as knowing ways to prevent poisoning exposures, is a vital component of basic first aid. An emergency medical responder should activate EMS for a patient who exhibits any signs or symptoms of a life-threatening condition (sleepiness, seizures, difficulty breathing, or vomiting) after exposure to a poison.

Poison is the kind of thing you're not supposed to touch
Old prescriptions, cleaning stuff or spider bites and such
If you swallowed something bad,
or think you took too much
Call the Poison Control Center Hotline
We're the people you can trust.

Source: American Association of Poison Control Centers

What to do if a poisoning occurs:

1. Remain calm
2. Call 9-1-1 if the patient is unconscious or not breathing; call the Poison Control Center if the patient is conscious
3. Have the following information available when you call:
   a. Patient's age and weight
   b. The container or bottle of the poison if available
   c. The time of the poison exposure
   d. The address where the poisoning occurred
4. Follow the instructions of the EMS dispatch operator or the PCC

Sources

American Association of Poison Control Centers www.aapcc.org

American Heart Association and the American National Red Cross (2010). Part 17: First Aid: 2010 American Heart Association and American Red Cross Guidelines for First Aid. *Circulation* 2010, 122:S93-S946. www.circulationaha.org

Bronstein, AC, et. al (2008). 2007 Annual Report of the American Association of Poison Control Centers National Poison Data System: 25th Annual Report, *Clinical Toxicology*, 46: 10, 927 – 1057.

Centers for Disease Control and Prevention, National Center for Injury Prevention and Control www.cdc.gov/HomeandRecreationalSafety/Poisoning/poisoning-factsheet.htm

National Capital Poison Center www.poison.org

National Institute on Drug Abuse
http://www.drugabuse.gov/publications/drugfacts-related-hospital-emergency-room-visits

Name: ______________________ Date: __________

Learning Activities

I. Multiple Choice

1. Most poisonings occur in the
   a. Home
   b. Workplace
   c. Hospital
   d. School

2. The general care for most ingested poisons includes
   a. Giving milk or water to drink
   b. Calling the PCC or 9-1-1
   c. Inducing vomiting
   d. All of the above

3. An emergency medical responder performs a primary assessment on a patient with a suspected ingested poison. The patient is unconscious and breathing. How should the EMR position this patient?
   a. In the supine position
   b. In the modified H.A.IN.E.S. recovery position
   c. In a position of comfort
   d. In a prone position with head turned to one side

4. To provide care for a patient suffering from an inhaled poison, such as carbon monoxide, the emergency medical responder should immediately
   a. Loosen any clothing around the patient's neck
   b. Move the patient into fresh air
   c. Begin artificial ventilations
   d. Call 9-1-1 or the PCC

5. Among those individuals who died from unintentional poisonings, which age group had the highest percentage of deaths?
   a. Children under the age of 6
   b. Children 6–12 years of age
   c. Adolescents 13–19 years of age
   d. Persons 20–59 years of age

6. Where would a poison control center most likely be located?
   a. In a public health department
   b. In an emergency department of a large medical center
   c. In a fire department
   d. All of the above

7. Signs and symptoms of ingested poisonings include all of the following except
   a. Body tremors
   b. Problems breathing
   c. Burns around and in the mouth
   d. Headache

8. When a patient is exposed to a poison, the emergency medical responder can often call the PCC to determine the appropriate care to administer. Which of the following signs and symptoms would indicate to the EMR that EMS should be called instead?
   a. The patient complains about chest pressure.
   b. The patient is acting out of character, in a violent manner.
   c. The patient is having trouble breathing.
   d. All of the above would indicate a call.

9. Sources of chemical poisonings include
   a. Mercury
   b. Lead
   c. Aluminum
   d. Both a and b

10. The most deadly form of food poisoning is
   a. Botulism
   b. Salmonella
   c. Shigella
   d. Escherichia coli (E. coli)

11. In a patient who has ingested a poison, vomiting should never be induced if which of the following situations is present?
   a. The patient is pregnant.
   b. The patient swallowed a corrosive substance.
   c. The patient has heart disease.
   d. All of the above are correct.

12. Carbon monoxide is a poisonous gas found in
   a. Fires
   b. Kerosene heaters
   c. Defective gas furnaces
   d. All of the above

13. A patient spills a dry chemical on his arm. The emergency medical responder should brush the chemical off using
   a. His bare hand
   b. His gloved hand
   c. A towel
   d. Both b and c

14. Of the following signs and symptoms, which one would alert the emergency medical responder that the patient is experiencing an overdose of a stimulant?
   a. Irritability
   b. Lethargy
   c. Incoherent speech
   d. Increased heart rate

15. When you arrive at the scene of an emergency, you suspect substance abuse. Which of the following would be a priority for the emergency medical responder?
    a. Summon more advanced medical personnel.
    b. Identify the exact substance and dose that was involved.
    c. Restrain the patient to prevent self-injury.
    d. Maintain the patient's body temperature.

16. A child who was bitten by a venomous snake was poisoned through which route?
    a. Inhalation
    b. Absorption
    c. Ingestion
    d. Injection

17. Oxycodone belongs to which category of medication?
    a. Narcotic
    b. Depressant
    c. Stimulants
    d. Hallucinogens

II. Short Answer

1. Identify the four ways through which poisons can enter the body.

    1.

    2.

    3.

    4.

2. When calling the poison control center for help with a suspected poisoning, what information should be provided?

3. To care for a patient who has come in contact with an absorbed poison, the emergency medical responder should rinse the skin for at least ________minutes.

4. Medications that reduce the inflammation produced by absorbed poisons are known as ______________________________drugs.

5. Medications that can dry up lesions and reduce the itching associated with absorbed poisons are known as ______________________________.

III. True or False

_______ 1. First aid for emergencies caused by substance abuse or overdose follows the same steps as for any poisoning.

_______ 2. Attempt to restrain a patient of suspected drug abuse who becomes agitated or threatening to prevent self-injury.

_______ 3. Immediately wash any affected areas that have come into contact with poison ivy, using soap and water.

_______ 4. If a poison has come in contact with a patient's eye, the eye should be flushed with clean water for at least 20 minutes.

_______ 5. Apply ice or a cold pack to the site of a bitten area immediately.

IV. Scenarios

Scenario 1

You and your husband are involved in a home remodeling project. Your husband has removed the kitchen cabinets and is preparing to strip the old paint, using a commercial paint stripping product. While pouring the solution out of the container, it slips from his hands and falls to the ground. Some of the solution splashes on his pants and burns his lower legs and feet. (Question 1 refers to scenario 1)

1. What should his wife should do in this situation?

Scenario 2

A 15-year-old girl is babysitting her 3-year-old brother. She leaves him playing in the family room in order to prepare a snack in the kitchen. When she returns, she finds her brother eating tablets from a bottle of aspirin spilled on the floor. (Questions 1–2 refer to Scenario 2.)

1. What is the first action that the girl should take?
   a. Call the child's doctor.
   b. Call the PCC.
   c. Make the child vomit.
   d. Give the child water to drink.

2. What could have been done to prevent this situation from happening?

Scenario 3

A family moved into an apartment during the month of January. The gas and electric were supposed to be turned on before the family moved in, however, that did not happen. The husband turned to the landlord for help in heating the apartment. The landlord gave the family a portable generator to use temporarily until the utilities were activated. The husband set the generator up inside the apartment, neglecting to vent the carbon monoxide fumes outside. The following morning, the landlord arrived at the apartment to check on the family. After he discovered all the family members lying unconscious on the living room floor, he called 9-1-1 and turned off the generator. (Questions 1–2 refer to this Scenario.)

1. As the emergency medical responder, what is your first priority when arriving on the scene?
   a. Make sure that the electric and gas companies are called
   b. Open the doors and windows in the apartment
   c. Make sure the scene is safe to enter
   d. Put on personal protective equipment

2. During the primary assessment, you find that the family members are unconscious, have a weak pulse, and are breathing about 4–5 times per minute. Your initial care would include
   a. Placing the patients in a modified H.A.IN.E.S. recovery position
   b. Administering CPR
   c. Administering ventilations
   d. Preventing the onset of shock

Scenario 4

A frantic neighbor is pounding on your door. She says that she cannot awaken her sleeping roommate. The neighbor remembers that earlier her roommate was complaining about having a severe headache and not being able to fall asleep. The neighbor saw her roommate take a handful of pills several hours ago but she isn't sure what she took and can't locate the pill container. When you enter the apartment, you see a woman lying supine on the couch. She isn't moving and she appears to have vomited recently. Her respiration rate is approximately six breaths per minute and very shallow and her pulse is 56 and weak. (Questions 1–2 refer to Scenario 4.)

1. When you check the woman's level of consciousness, you find her to be unresponsive. What should you do next?

2. Prioritize the steps that you would take to care for this patient.

V. Web-Based Exercise (Extra Credit Assignment)

There are currently 62 poison control centers located throughout the United States and in Puerto Rico. Go to the American Association of Poison Control Centers website (www.aapcc.org).

Select a state ______________________________.

1. Where are the poison control centers located in that state?

2. How many states do **NOT** have a poison control center and are served by another state? Identify each state and name the state that provides coverage.

16 Environmental Emergencies

Expanded Chapter Content

- Heat-Related Emergencies
  - Care for Heat Stroke
- Cold-Related Emergencies
  - Care for Frostbite
- Anaphylaxis and the Epi-Pen Auto Injector
- Care for Snake Bites
- Care for Jellyfish Stings

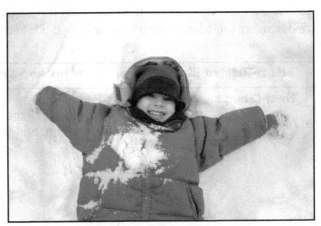

Chapter Significance

As an emergency medical responder, you may be called upon to assist a patient who is suffering from extremes in outside temperatures (*hyperthermia* or *hypothermia*). While each of these conditions begins with mild signs and symptoms, each can progress into life-threatening conditions if they are not properly evaluated and treated.

This chapter also discusses environmental emergencies such as various types of insect and animal bites. One of the most important aspects of providing care to a patient who has been stung by an insect or bitten by an animal is to assess the patient for signs and symptoms of *anaphylaxis*, a respiratory emergency leading to respiratory arrest within about 10 minutes of being stung or bitten. In this situation, the primary responsibility of an emergency medical responder is to activate EMS and administer the *epinephrine auto-injector* if one is available.

CHECK ▪ CALL ▪ CARE

Heat-Related Emergencies and Care for Heat Stroke

The human body is well equipped to withstand extremes in temperature. Under normal circumstances, its mechanisms for regulating body temperature work well. However, when the body is overwhelmed, life-threatening medical problems can develop.

Heat-Related Illnesses

There are three main types of illnesses that can develop when people are overexposed to heat: ***heat cramps, heat exhaustion,*** and ***heat stroke***. Heat cramps are the mildest form but, if left untreated with continuing exposure, may progress to heat exhaustion and finally heat stroke. Heat stroke is associated with a high mortality rate. When the body temperature is excessively high, it causes the brain and other vital organs to fail. All three conditions are caused by excessive loss of body fluids (*dehydration*) and *electrolytes*.

Heat-Related Illnesses	**Signs and Symptoms**	**Care**
1. **Heat Cramps**	• Painful muscle spasms affecting primarily the arms, calves, abdomen, and back	• Rest in a cool place. • Stretching, icing, and massaging painful arm or leg muscles may be helpful. • Exercise should not be resumed until all symptoms have been resolved. • Give cool water or an electrolyte-carbohydrate beverage to drink. • Do **NOT** give salt tablets or salt water.
2. **Heat Exhaustion**—usually caused by a combination of exercise-induced heat and fluid and electrolytes lost in sweat.	• *Skin:* pale or ashen, cool, moist; heavy sweating • *Vital Signs:* normal or slightly elevated temperature, rapid breathing and pulse • *Behaviors:* weakness, tiredness, dizziness, headache, thirst, nausea and vomiting • May or may not have muscle cramps	Take steps to cool the body and replenish fluids and electrolytes. • Move the patient to a cool environment (shady or air-conditioned). • Remove as much clothing as possible. • If fully conscious and not vomiting, provide cool fluids, preferably containing carbohydrates and electrolytes. Instruct to drink slowly. Avoid alcoholic or caffeinated beverages. • Cool down using one of these methods: Apply cool wet towels or cloths to the back of the neck, underarms, wrists, groins, and ankles. Spray water on the patient with a spray bottle then fan the patient. If no improvement or the condition worsens within 30 minutes, call 9-1-1.

Heat-Related Illnesses	Signs and Symptoms	♥ Care
3. **Heat Stroke**—includes all the signs and symptoms of heat exhaustion plus central nervous system involvement.	• *Skin:* flushed, hot, dry; no sweating. • *Vital Signs:* temperature often above 104° F., rapid heart rate and rapid, shallow breathing • *Altered mental status* ranging from dizziness, fainting, confusion and possible seizures • Nausea and vomiting	• Call 9-1-1. • Move to a cool environment (shady or air-conditioned). • Remove as much clothing as possible. • Cool the patient quickly by any means: Apply ice or cold packs to areas of the body where large blood vessels are close to the surface. Place a barrier between the cold source and the skin. Spray water with a hose or spray bottle and fan the patient. • Do not give the patient anything to eat or drink if they are not fully conscious. • Monitor the ABCs while awaiting EMS • Be prepared to give artificial ventilations or perform CPR, if necessary.

*** The American Red Cross states that the most important action by a first aid provider is to begin immediate cooling of the patient, preferably by immersing the patient up to their chin in cold water.

Cold-Related Illnesses and Care for Frostbite

There are two main types of cold-related illnesses: ***frostbite*** and ***hypothermia.***
Frostbite is a condition in which body tissues freeze. The tissues most commonly affected are areas of the skin exposed to cold with the poorest circulation (face, hands, and feet). The signs and symptoms of frostbite vary, depending on whether the frostbite is *superficial* or *deep*.

Care for Frostbite:

- Remove the patient from the cold environment and prevent hypothermia.
- Remove any wet clothing and jewelry. Do **NOT** massage any affected areas.
- Get the patient to a medical facility as quickly as possible.
- For a minor frostbite injury, the American Red Cross recommends skin-to-skin contact to rewarm the body part; for a more serious injury, immerse the body part in warm water, no hotter than 105° F. If you don't have a thermometer, test the water with your hand—if the temperature is uncomfortable for you, it is too hot.
- If you are far from a medical facility and there is no chance the frostbitten part will refreeze, you can rewarm the affected body part by placing it in warm water (100–105° F.) until it turns red or feels warm.
- Protect frostbitten areas on the hands or feet by placing gauze between the fingers or toes and wrapping them loosely with dry, sterile dressings.

Scenario: A few years ago, a 20-month-old girl slipped out of her family's home on a cold November day in Fullerton, California. Shortly thereafter, she was found floating face down in 52° water in the family's swimming pool. A 9-1-1 call was placed by the mother and two policemen arrived within several minutes and began CPR until EMS arrived and transported the child to the hospital. In the emergency room, the child was wrapped in a heating blanket and CPR was continued. After an hour of performing CPR without any vital signs, the child was pronounced dead. Approximately 40 minutes later, a detective was photographing the child's body when he thought he saw her chest move. He thought the movements were just muscle spasms except they were coming with regular frequency. He called in the doctor and nurses who examined the child and found that she had a pulse and was breathing! How could this have happened? A theory as to why this occurred is that the heating blanket had not been turned off when the child was pronounced dead. The child's core body temperature was probably still in the mid to upper 80s—not warm enough to "jumpstart" her heart and breathing. It took another 45 minutes or so for the child's core body temperature to reach a normal level (98.6° F), and when that happened, her pulse and breathing returned.

When a patient suffers severe *hypothermia*, care (such as CPR) must be prolonged because the patient's body won't respond until normal body temperature is reached. Since severe hypothermia reduces the vital organ's oxygen requirements, once the patient is resuscitated, brain damage may be minimal. This child suffered no brain damage from the severe and prolonged hypothermia.

Hypothermia refers to a condition in which the body temperature drops below 95° F, due to cold exposure. The patient's condition can range from mild to moderate to severe and life-threatening. The urgency of treatment depends upon the length of exposure and the patient's body temperature.

Care for hypothermia is directed at two objectives:

1. Gradually rewarm the patient.
2. Prevent further heat loss.
   - Move the patient to a heated environment.
   - Call 9-1-1 or local emergency number.
   - Perform a primary assessment; check for pulse and breathing for 30–45 seconds instead of 10 seconds.
   - Remove any wet clothing and dry the patient.
   - Cover the patient with dry clothing, if available, and warm blankets.
   - If available, apply hot water bottles or commercial heat packs to the underarms and groins. Place a barrier between the patient's skin and the heat source.
   - If alert and able to swallow, provide the patient with warm nonalcoholic, decaffeinated liquids to drink.

Expanded Chapter Content

Anaphylaxis and the Epi-pen auto injector.

In retrospective studies, 18–35% of patients having signs and symptoms of anaphylaxis required a second dose of epinephrine because symptoms persisted or progressed after the first dose. Because of the difficulty in making a diagnosis of anaphylaxis and the potential harm from epinephrine if the diagnosis is incorrect, first aid providers are advised to seek medical assistance if symptoms persist rather than routinely administer a second dose of epinephrine. The American Red Cross guidelines state that in unusual circumstances, such as if signs of *anaphylaxis* persist after a few minutes, EMS is delayed and state law permits, a second dose of epinephrine (through the Epi-pen auto injector) should be given.

Scenario: A Swanton township man died after he was stung once in the neck by a bee or wasp while he was putting chickens into a coop at his home. The man was pronounced dead about 10 minutes after being stung. Following the autopsy, the coroner's office stated that the man died of an acute anaphylactic reaction.

- Check the label on the **Epi-pen** to verify that it is for the patient.
- Ensure that the expiration date has not passed (Figure 16.1)
- Make sure that the medication is clear; do not use if it is cloudy or discolored.
- Make sure that the patient has not already taken a dose of epinephrine. Do not administer a second dose unless instructed to do so by EMS personnel.

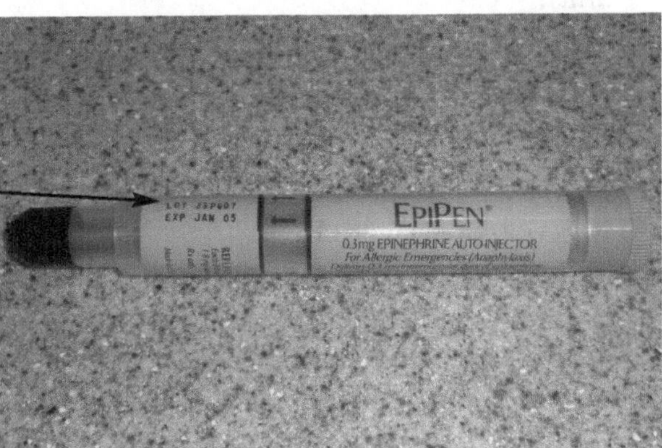

Figure 16.1

Anaphylaxis and Epinephrine Auto-injector

The primary responsibility of the emergency medical responder is to recognize that the patient is experiencing an anaphylactic reaction and take immediate action. Follow these steps to care for an anaphylactic reaction:

- Verify that the patient is experiencing an anaphylactic reaction through statements made by the patient or family members, and the signs and symptoms that you observe.
- Activate 9-1-1 immediately.

Epinephrine is a medication which is used to decrease bronchospasm and keep the airways open. It is most effective when given by injection into the muscle. If an epinephrine auto-injector is available (**Epi-pen**), follow these steps:

It is preferable for the patient to self-administer the injection. However, depending on the severity of the patient's signs and symptoms, he or she may not be able to do so. Emergency medical responders should be able to administer the medication if the patient is unable to do so since it has been prescribed by a physician, and state law permits it. In this situation, the emergency medical responder should follow these steps:

Step 1

- Remove the gray cap from the auto-injector (Figure 16.2).

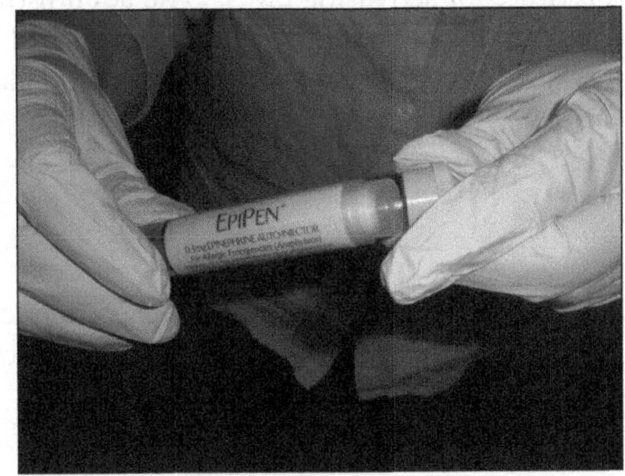

Figure 16.2

Step 2

- Find the middle of the outer aspect of the thigh for the injection site (may also use the upper arm).
- Grasp the auto-injector firmly in your fist and remove the safety cap. Do not place your fingers under the tip of the pen.
- Hold the auto-injector at a 90° angle to the injection site (Figure 16.3).

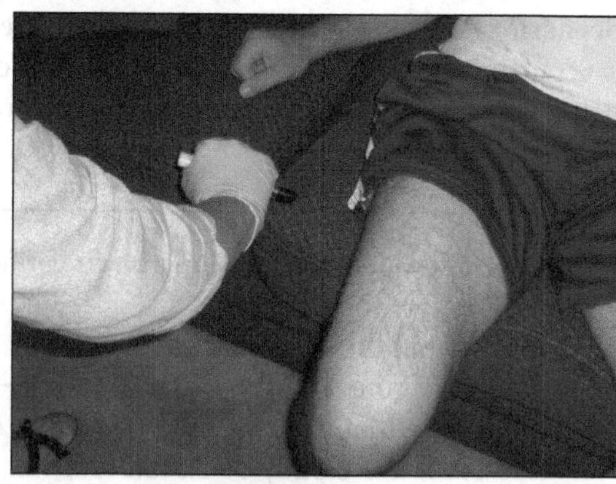

Figure 16.3

Step 3

- Quickly and firmly, jab the auto-injector straight into the injection site (through clothing if necessary). You will hear a "click" which lets you know that the needle has been engaged and the medication has been released.
- Hold the auto-injector in place for 10 seconds (Figure 16.4).

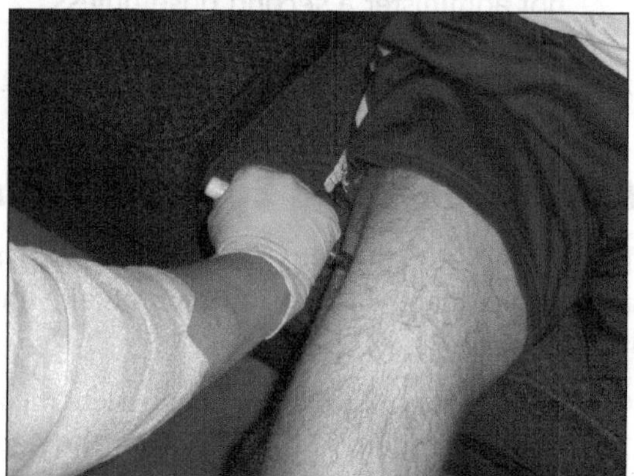

Figure 16.4

Step 4

- Remove the auto-injector and massage the injection site for several seconds (Figure 16.5).
- Place the auto-injector inside a container to prevent injuries or give it to EMS personnel.
- Monitor vital signs until EMS arrives.

Remember that the use of the Epi-pen is not a substitute for activating EMS. The administration of epinephrine will help slow the progression of respiratory distress but the effects of the medication are short acting.

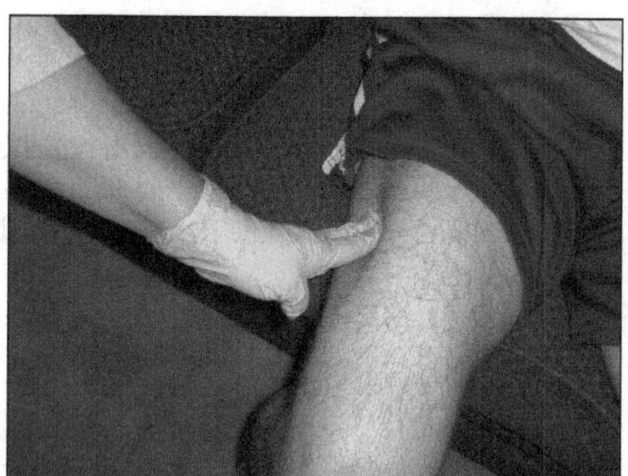

Figure 16.5

Source

American Heart Association and the American National Red Cross (2010). Part 17: First Aid: 2010 American Heart Association and American Red Cross Guidelines for First Aid. *Circulation* 2010, 122: S934-S946. www.circulationaha.org

Expanded Chapter Content

Care for Snake Bites

Irrigate human and animal bites with copious amounts of water. This irrigation has been shown to prevent rabies from animal bites and bacterial infection.

All snake bites should be irrigated with large amounts of clean water followed by the application of a pressure immobilization bandage. The bandage should be snug enough to slow the dissemination of the venom by slowing lymph flow. Pressure should be comfortably tight and snug but allows a finger to be slipped under it.

Jellyfish Stings

First aid for jellyfish stings consists of two important actions: preventing further nematocyst discharge and pain relief. After the stingers/tentacles are removed, soak the affected body part in hot water (at least 113° F), or as hot as the patient can tolerate for at least 20 minutes or until the pain persists. If hot water is not readily available, pack the extremity in hot sand.

Name: ______________________________ Date: ______________

Learning Activities

I. Multiple Choice

1. The majority of heat loss from the body is through the process of
   a. Respiration
   b. Radiation
   c. Conduction
   d. Convection

2. Emergency care for frostbite includes
   a. Massaging the affected areas vigorously to restore circulation
   b. Running hot water over the affected area for 10 minutes
   c. Removing wet clothing and jewelry from the affected area
   d. Applying direct heat, such as a heating pad, to rapidly unthaw the frozen tissue

3. What is the first action to take for a patient with a suspected heat-related illness who begins to lose consciousness?
   a. Cool the patient using wet sheets, towels, or cold packs.
   b. Cool the body by applying rubbing alcohol.
   c. Call 9-1-1.
   d. Both a and c are first actions.

4. Caring for a person who is experiencing heat cramps should include
   a. Giving salt tablets
   b. Activating EMS
   c. Resting in a cool place
   d. All of the above

5. Emergency care for a patient of hypothermia should include
   a. Vigorously rubbing the patient's extremities
   b. Soaking the patient in warm water
   c. Removing wet clothing
   d. All of the above

6. A patient was swimming in the ocean off the eastern coast of the United States and was stung by a jellyfish. As an emergency medical responder, what should you do first?
   a. Flush the injured part with vinegar for 30 seconds.
   b. Apply meat tenderizer to the area.
   c. Rinse the area with fresh water.
   d. Apply aluminum sulfate to the area.

7. The signs and symptoms of heat exhaustion include
   a. Deep breathing
   b. Cool, moist, pale skin
   c. Loss of consciousness
   d. High blood pressure

8. What is the first priority in providing emergency care for a patient experiencing heat cramps?
   a. Forcing fluids at frequent intervals
   b. Moving the patient out of the heat
   c. Reducing cramps with light massage
   d. Apply wet cool cloths to the cramping muscle

9. Signs and symptoms of anaphylaxis include
   a. Rash or hives
   b. Difficulty breathing
   c. Tight feeling in the throat or chest
   d. All of the above

10. A characteristic "bulls-eye" rash is characteristic of which disease?
    a. Lyme disease
    b. Rocky Mountain spotted fever
    c. Erlichiosis
    d. Babesia infection

11. When the stinger/tentacles of a jellyfish have been removed, the best method to reduce the pain of the sting is to
    a. Give the patient two Tylenol tablets
    b. Apply an ice pack to the area for 20 minutes
    c. Immerse the area in hot water for 20 minutes
    d. Apply a pressure bandage over the area

12. First aid for a snake bite usually includes
    a. Cleaning the wound with soap and water
    b. Applying a tourniquet on the bitten extremity above the bite
    c. Applying a suction device over the wound
    d. Cutting in the shape of an X over the wound

13. The best way to remove an embedded tick is to
    a. Cover the tick with a cotton ball soaked in alcohol
    b. Touch the tick with a hot match
    c. Grab the tick with your fingers and pull gently
    d. Pull the tick out gently with tweezers

II. Short Answer

1. Explain why infants and elderly individuals are at an increased risk for hypothermia.

2. Hypothermia is defined as a core body temperature below ________ ° F.

3. What is the rationale for wrapping a patient's bitten extremity with an elastic roller bandage as an emergency treatment for snakebite?

4. A bluebottle, or Portuguese man-of-war, jellyfish sting should be flushed with ________________.

5. A patient who has been bitten by an animal or a human may require a ____________ booster.

III. True or False

_______ 1. Shivering is observed in patients suffering from severe hypothermia.

_______ 2. To prevent heat-related illnesses, wear dark clothing when working outside in hot weather.

_______ 3. A person does not have to be exposed to below freezing temperatures for hypothermia to occur.

IV. Scenarios

Scenario 1
It was the first week of football spring training with the heat index above 105° F. The team has been working hard all day. The athletic trainer noticed that one of the players suddenly walked off the field and then seemed to collapse. When she approached the player, she noted that he was awake but having trouble speaking clearly and coherently; his skin was hot and dry to the touch. (Questions 1–3 refer to Scenario 1.)

1. Based on the patient's signs and symptoms, what heat-related illness is this patient experiencing?

2. Identify the information **in the scenario** that would lead you to suspect that this was the problem. (Remember to **check** the environment and **check** the patient.)

3. Describe the actions you would take to **care** for this patient.

Scenario 2

You have been involved in a search for a lost 6-year-old boy. The search is now into its third day. The child became lost when he wandered away from his mountain campsite. He has already spent two nights in the wilderness in cold, rainy weather. When the child is discovered, he is shivering and disoriented. His clothing is wet and his face and hands are cold to the touch. (Questions 1–3 refer to Scenario 2.)

1. What would you call this medical emergency?

2. What information from the scenario helped you to arrive at a decision regarding what might be wrong with the child?

3. Based on the above, what care do you provide to this child?

Scenario 3

It is late afternoon, and your team is finishing its third match of the beach volleyball tournament. It has been a really hot day, with temperatures in the 90s. Suddenly a teammate collapses. She does not appear to be fully conscious, but is breathing rapidly. You notice that her skin is very warm, sunburned, and moist. Her pulse is very fast. She is unable to get up from the ground. (Questions 1–3 refer to Scenario 3.)

1. What heat-related condition do you think this patient is experiencing?

2. Identify the information provided in the scenario that you used to support your answer to question 1.

3. As an emergency medical responder, how would you care for this patient?

17 Behavioral Emergencies

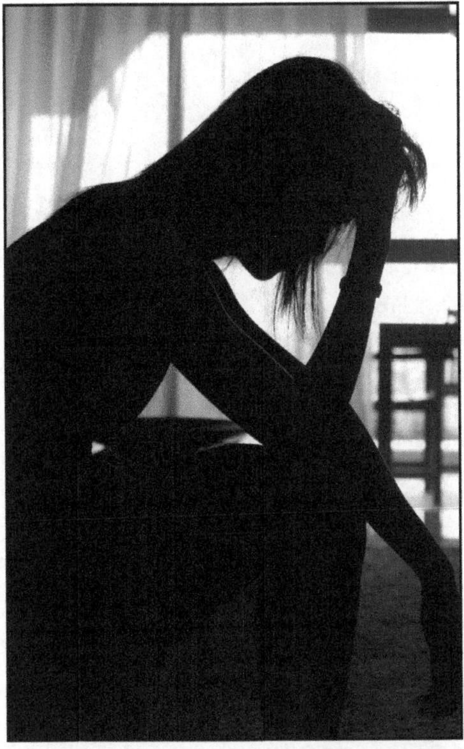

Chapter Significance

The focus of this chapter is behavioral emergencies, which present special challenges for the emergency medical responder. Most emergency medical responders are not adequately trained to handle a behavioral emergency, thereby putting themselves at risk. If you encounter a patient who is experiencing a behavioral emergency, your immediate action would be to activate 9-1-1. As you learned in Chapter 2, the most important responsibility of the emergency medical responder is to ensure the safety of yourself and any bystanders; do not put yourself in harm's way.

CHECK ▪ CALL ▪ CARE

Name: ______________________ Date: __________

Learning Activities

I. Multiple Choice

1. The definition of a behavioral emergency is any behavior that
   a. Can cause harm to the patient
   b. Threatens to harm bystanders or family members
   c. Is intolerable or unacceptable
   d. Involves a weapon

2. Causes of a behavioral emergency include
   a. Drugs or alcohol
   b. Lack of oxygen to the brain
   c. Head injuries
   d. All of the above

3. A mental illness in which the patient hears voices is known as
   a. Bipolar disorder
   b. Excited delirium syndrome
   c. Paranoia
   d. Schizophrenia

4. A mental illness characterized by periods of depression alternating with periods of hyperexcitability is
   a. Schizophrenia
   b. Bipolar disorder
   c. Schizophrenia
   d. Self-mutilation

5. An unhealthy coping mechanism to deal with negative emotions such as tension, anger, and frustration is
   a. Clinical depression
   b. Self-mutilation
   c. Phobias
   d. Anxiety disorder

6. How can an emergency medical responder establish rapport with a patient who is experiencing a behavioral emergency?
   a. Speak directly to the patient.
   b. Avoid making eye contact with the patient.
   c. Touch the patient on the shoulder.
   d. Tell the patient that everything will be fine.

7. An emergency medical responder may place a patient in restraints for which of the following reasons?
   a. The patient is unresponsive.
   b. The patient is refusing care.
   c. The patient is thrashing and kicking.
   d. The patient is shouting for help.

8. An emergency medical responder arrives at the scene of an emergency where the patient is threatening to commit suicide. Which of the following actions would be most appropriate?
   a. Call the patient's bluff about the threat to commit suicide.
   b. Deny that the patient wants to commit suicide.
   c. Call for additional trained personnel and do not approach the scene.
   d. Tell the patient that he or she is too scared to commit suicide.

II. Short Answer

1. An irrational fear of objects or events that are usually harmless is known as a ________________.

2. An intentional act to end one's life is called ______________________.

3. Any form of sexual contact against a person's will, often through coercion or threat, is called ____________________________.

4. Another term for bipolar disorder is ___________________________________.

III. True or False

_______ 1. A person experiencing a behavioral emergency has control over his feelings.

_______ 2. Assume that a patient with a behavioral emergency has an altered mental status.

_______ 3. It can be very difficult to provide care to a patient who is paranoid.

_______ 4. The 15- to 24-year-old age group is at highest risk for death by suicide.

_______ 5. Elderly individuals are at a higher risk than the general population for suicide.

_______ 6. If a patient is experiencing hallucinations, the emergency medical responder should play along with the patient.

_______ 7. If the patient has a weapon, the emergency medical responder should not enter the scene.

_______ 8. The emergency medical responder may restrain a violent, combative patient as part of the standing orders.

IV. Scenarios

Scenario 1

You are home alone when the doorbell rings. When you answer the door, a man and woman are on the doorstep extremely agitated and crying. The woman tells you that they were visiting with her father next door when he abruptly left the room. After a few minutes, they heard what sounded like a gunshot. They called the father's name, but he didn't answer so they ran to your house. (Questions 1–2 refer to Scenario 1.)

1. Based on this situation, what is the first action for you to take?

2. The woman is very upset and wants to enter the house to check on her father. What should you do in this situation?

Scenario 2

You are seated at a restaurant eating dinner. Suddenly a middle-aged woman, dressed in a provocative manner, walks into the restaurant. You notice her odd behavior as she begins moving from table to table, talking quickly and excitedly and reciting verses from the Bible. The patrons are uncomfortable and afraid; they don't know what to say to the woman. Occasionally she begins singing in a loud voice, telling everyone she is Madonna. Attempts to remove her by restaurant personnel are futile. (Questions 1–4 refer to Scenario 2.)

1. As an emergency medical responder, what is your priority in this situation?

2. While awaiting the arrival of EMS, how can you establish rapport with a patient experiencing a behavioral emergency?

3. What steps can you take to calm a patient experiencing a behavioral emergency?

4. When EMS arrives, the patient becomes combative and starts throwing things at the EMS personnel. A decision was made to restrain the patient. What are safety and legal issues for the use of restraints on a patient?

Unit 6

Trauma Emergencies

18 Shock

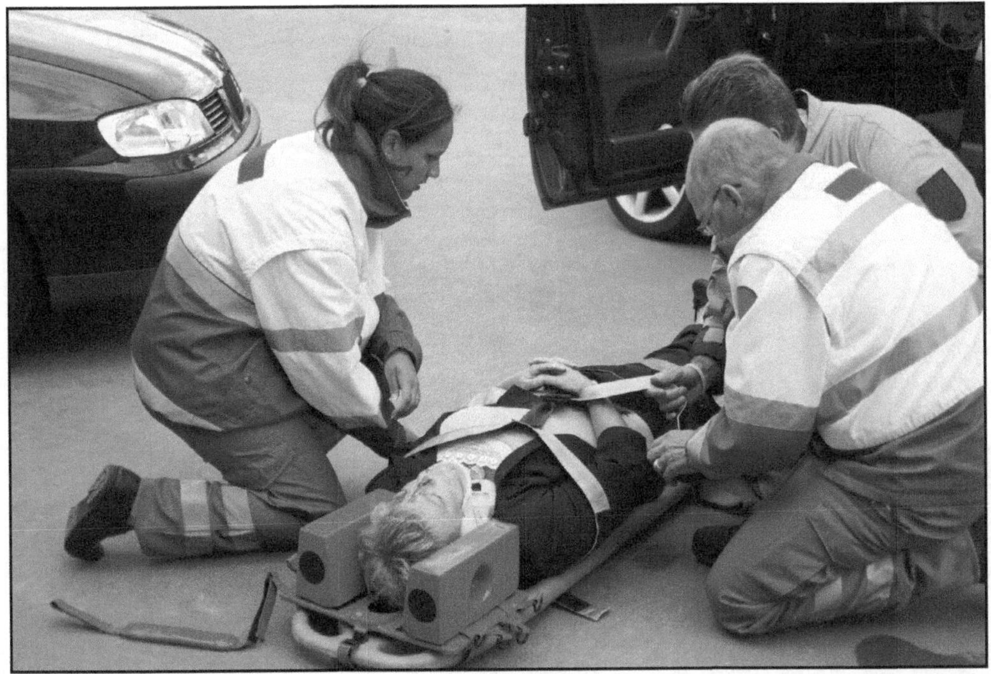

Chapter Significance

A patient who has suffered a serious medical emergency or injury may develop shock as a consequence of the situation. Shock is caused by a collapse of the circulatory system and its inability to supply vital organs with oxygen-rich blood. Regardless of the cause of shock, the outcome is the same. As the emergency medical responder is conducting a primary assessment to evaluate the patient for a life-threatening illness or injury, he or she must also recognize the signs and symptoms of shock and take the appropriate measures to minimize the occurrence of shock. Shock disrupts the perfusion of vital organs, causing them to die.

CHECK ▪ CALL ▪ CARE

Name: ______________________________ Date: ______________

Learning Activities

I. Multiple Choice

1. An early sign of shock is
   a. Apprehension and anxiety
   b. Drowsiness and confusion
   c. Shallow and slow breathing
   d. Slow pulse and low blood pressure

2. What would be the best method of positioning a patient who is showing signs of shock as a result of a spinal injury?
   a. Lying on the back with legs elevated
   b. Lying flat on the back
   c. In the modified H.A.IN.E.S. recovery position
   d. Lying on the back with the head raised 45° degrees

3. The skin changes that are characteristic of shock are caused by
   a. Damage to the temperature control center in the brain
   b. Shunting of blood away from the skin to vital organs
   c. Reduced heat production by the body
   d. Slowing of the heart's pumping action

4. Which of the following actions would not be appropriate for an emergency medical responder to do for a patient experiencing shock?
   a. Cover the patient with a blanket.
   b. Take steps to minimize blood loss.
   c. Give the patient a drink.
   d. Administer oxygen if it is available, and you are trained to do so.

5. Of the following statements, which one most accurately describes shock in children?
   a. Early signs of shock occur sooner than usual because of their small size.
   b. Hypovolemic shock requires a larger amount of blood loss in children.
   c. Children are less susceptible for the development of shock than adults.
   d. Children's bodies are better able to compensate for some factors that lead to shock.

II. Short Answer

1. Another name for shock is ____________________, a decrease in the amount of oxygenated blood being circulated to vital organs and body tissues.

2. In a healthy body, what three conditions must be necessary in order to maintain adequate blood flow?

3. The type of shock caused by severe blood loss is called ________________ shock.

4. List the four major types of shock and the causes of each type.

Type of Shock	Causes

5. Explain why the early signs and symptoms of shock are absent in young children.

III. Scenario

In the early morning, your neighbor lady runs over to your house screaming that her husband has severe chest pain. When you enter her house, you see an elderly man sitting on the sofa rubbing his chest. His skin is moist and ashen. His respirations are labored and rapid and his heart rate is elevated. He looks very anxious and apprehensive. (Questions 1–3 refer to Scenario 1.)

1. You suspect that this patient may be going into shock. What type of shock might this man be experiencing?

2. What information from the scenario led you to suspect that the patient may be exhibiting early signs and symptoms of shock?

3. List the care that you, as an emergency medical responder, should provide to this patient.

19 Bleeding and Trauma

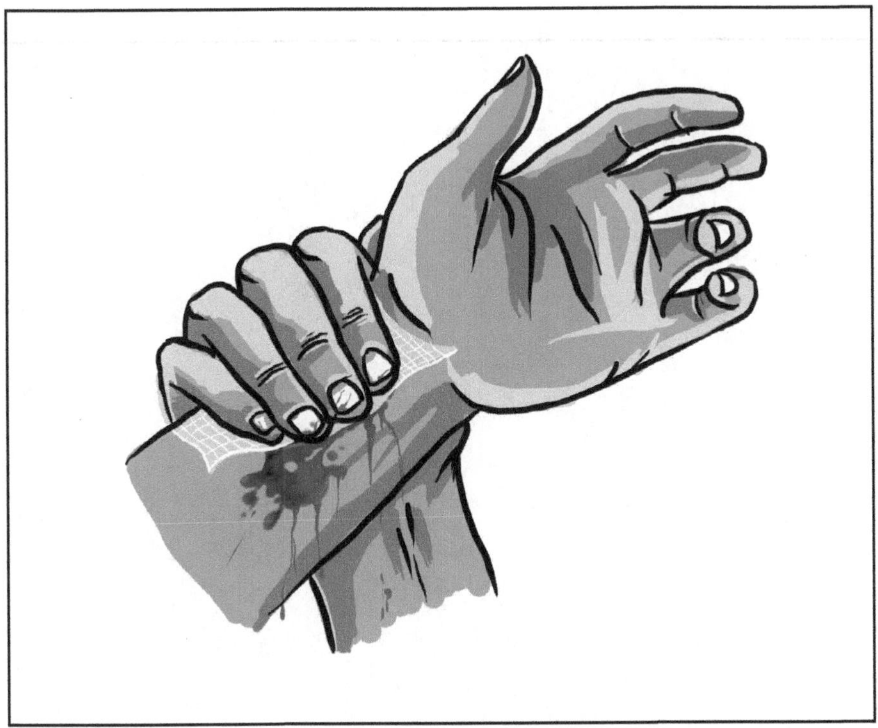

Chapter Significance

One of the primary responsibilities of an emergency medical responder in any situation is to identify and care for conditions that are potentially life-threatening. A patient who loses a large amount of blood within a short period of time (*hemorrhage*) can develop shock or die from the injuries without immediate care.

Bleeding results from injuries to arteries, capillaries, or veins and can be described as being either external or internal. Both external and internal bleeding can result in shock and death. In this chapter, you will learn how to identify and care for bleeding as a result of injuries to various

CHECK ▪ CALL ▪ CARE

blood vessels. As an emergency medical responder, you will learn how to control severe external bleeding through the application of direct pressure and the application of a pressure bandage. The amount of pressure applied and the time the pressure is held are the most important factors affecting successful control of bleeding. The pressure must be firm and maintained for a long period of time.

Other methods to control bleeding such as the use of a tourniquet, elevation of the body part above the level of the heart, applying pressure at an arterial pressure point, and the administration of hemostatic agents are also addressed.

Name: ______________________________ Date: ______________

Learning Activities

I. Multiple Choice

1. The first action to take in controlling bleeding from an open wound is to
   a. Flush the wound with running water
   b. Wrap the wound with an elastic bandage
   c. Apply pressure to the wound with your fingers or hand
   d. Elevate the wound above the level of the heart

2. Checking the patient for internal and external bleeding is performed during the
   a. Scene size-up
   b. Primary assessment
   c. Physical examination
   d. SAMPLE history

3. An emergency medical responder has applied a pressure bandage over a patient's laceration to the lower leg. What should the EMR do next if bleeding continues, soaking through the dressing and bandage?
   a. Apply manual pressure over the femoral artery.
   b. Add new dressings and bandages on top of the blood soaked bandage.
   c. Apply a tourniquet to the leg above the wound.
   d. Remove the soiled dressing and bandage and apply new ones.

4. An emergency medical responder recognizes bleeding from an artery because arterial bleeding is
   a. Slow and stops quickly
   b. Steady and oozing
   c. Fast and spurting
   d. Slow and hard to control

5. The best way for an emergency medical responder to control bleeding from a nosebleed is
   a. Place an ice pack on the patient's neck
   b. Pack the nostrils with cotton gauze
   c. Pinch the nostrils together
   d. Apply pressure to the bridge of the nose

6. Which of the following is characteristic of venous bleeding?
   a. It is bright red in color.
   b. It flows steadily.
   c. It spurts from a wound.
   d. It is difficult for the blood to form a clot.

7. How can an emergency medical responder protect oneself from disease transmission when caring for a patient who is bleeding?
   a. Wear disposable gloves.
   b. Wash hands thoroughly for 30 seconds after providing care.
   c. Use an alcohol-based hand sanitizer after providing care.
   d. Wear two pair of disposable gloves.

8. Which type of dressing is appropriate to use for a patient with a sucking chest wound?
   a. Trauma dressing
   b. Occlusive dressing
   c. Adhesive dressing
   d. Elastic dressing

9. You are attempting to control external bleeding. Which of the following steps should you do first?
   a. Apply direct pressure to the wound.
   b. Check for circulation beyond the injury.
   c. Cover the wound with a dressing.
   d. Secure the dressing with a roller bandage.

II. Short Answer

1. The loss of a large amount of blood over a short period of time is called ________________.

2. What is meant by the term *Golden Hour?*

3. Define the medical term *perfusion*.

4. Define the medical term *tourniquet*.

   Under what situation would a tourniquet be appropriate to use?

5. Define the term *hemostatic agent*.

6. What is a pressure point?

   Name the two pressure points that can be used to control external bleeding.

7. List the signs and symptoms an emergency medical responder would see in a patient with severe internal bleeding.

8. What is the most important action you can take for a patient who is bleeding internally?

III. True or False

_______ 1. If direct pressure alone does not stop bleeding from an open wound on the arm, the next step is to apply pressure over the brachial artery.

_______ 2. A pressure bandage has been applied too loosely if the person can wiggle the fingers or toes on the injured extremity.

_______ 3. The use of a tourniquet is a routine part of controlling severe external bleeding.

_______ 4. A special type of dressing that does not allow air to pass through is called an occlusive dressing.

_______ 5. A triangular bandage can be used to make a sling.

_______ 6. Capillary bleeding is the easiest type of bleeding to control.

_______ 7. The characteristic black and blue mark seen in a contusion is a sign of internal bleeding.

_______ 8. Serious internal bleeding can be controlled by applying cold packs over the injured area.

_______ 9. If an injury involves a hand or foot, it is acceptable to cover the fingers or toes with a pressure bandage.

_______ 10. A hemostatic agent is a product that thins the blood.

_______ 11. To control bleeding, it is appropriate to elevate a painful, deformed extremity above the level of the heart.

IV. Scenario

Scenario 1

While at an off-campus party to celebrate the start of a new school year, you witness a fight break out between two party-goers. Suddenly someone is pushed through a plate glass window onto the ground. You immediately approach the patient and see blood squirting from his arm, with a piece of glass sticking out of the wound. (Questions 1–4 refer to Scenario 1.)

1. Based on the information provided, this patient is experiencing ___________ bleeding.
   a. Arterial
   b. Capillary
   c. Venous
   d. Internal

2. The most important action for you to take initially is to
   a. Apply continuous pressure over the wound
   b. Find a piece of clothing or a shoelace to tie tightly around the arm
   c. Make sure EMS has been activated
   d. Pull the glass out of the wound

3. The bleeding appears to have slowed down, but you notice the patient's skin has become cool, pale, and sweaty. What do these signs mean to you?
   a. Sweating is a normal reaction to the stress of being injured.
   b. The patient's body is trying to compensate for a serious injury.
   c. The patient is recovering from the traumatic injury.
   d. The patient needs fluids to drink from excessive fluid loss.

4. While awaiting the arrival of EMS, what would be the most appropriate position for this patient?
   a. Flat on his back
   b. On his back with legs raised
   c. Lying on his side
   d. Sitting up with the arm elevated

Scenario 2

A 35-year-old man was working on a property near Cleveland, thinning trees for the homeowners on the back of their property. He was using a chain saw to cut down a tree when the tree fell on top of him. The bottom half of the tree, which was 1.5 feet in diameter, pinched and severed his leg just below the knee when the tree came down. The man called 9-1-1 and explained that the tree, not the chain saw, had severed his leg. "A tree fell on my leg," he told 911 dispatchers. "It's completely severed." (Questions 1–4 refer to Scenario 2.)

1. If you were the first person to arrive on the scene, what would be your priority?

2. As an emergency medical responder, you examine the patient's leg and notice that it is bleeding profusely. What method would you use to control this patient's bleeding?

3. What condition is this patient at risk for since he lost a large amount of blood?

4. Outline the steps you would take to provide care for this patient.

Scenario 3

You arrive at a scene where a man is lying on the sidewalk. One leg appears to be bleeding. He is very pale and is breathing heavily, but he is conscious and able to speak, although he appears to be in pain. When you approach him, he waves you off and yells at you to go away. When you explain who you are and that you are trained and want to help him, he says he doesn't want any help. He tells you that his friends will take care of him yet you see no one around. (Questions 1–5 refer to Scenario 3.)

1. Based on the information in the scenario, what conditions do you think the man is suffering from?

2. What do you think about this man's *competence* (refer to Chapter 3)?

3. The man has refused treatment, even though he has a serious injury. Are you allowed to treat this man as an emergency medical responder? Provide rationale for your answer.

4. If you were able to treat this man, what care would you provide?

5. If the man continued to refuse care, what can you do as an emergency medical responder to protect yourself from a lawsuit charging *abandonment*?

Scenario 4
While hiking, a man strays from the path in search of more challenging terrain. He loses his footing on loose rocks and slides approximately 50 feet down a rocky slope. When you arrive, you notice that he is bleeding profusely from a deep laceration on his lower leg. He is pale, sweating, his skin feels cool, and he complains of feeling dizzy. (Questions 1–3 refer to Scenario 4.)

1. Based on this man's signs and symptoms, what condition do you think is occurring?

2. Describe the steps that you would take to control bleeding.

3. What steps can be taken to minimize the condition listed in question 1?

20 Soft Tissue Injuries

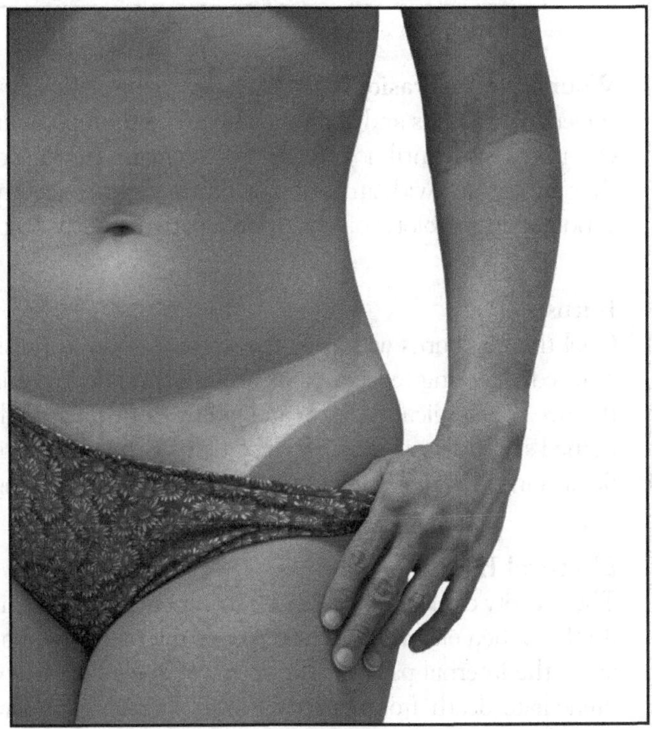

© Amy Walters, 2009. Used under license from Shutterstock, Inc.

Expanded Chapter Content

- Wounds and Abrasions
- Burns
- Electrical Injuries
- Chemical Burns

Chapter Significance

This chapter focuses primarily on specific types of injuries to layers of the skin, called soft-tissue injuries. Soft-tissue injuries include *closed wounds* such as bruises and *open wounds* such as *abrasions*, *lacerations*, *puncture/penetration*, *avulsion/amputation*, and *crush injuries*. Often, these injuries are minor; at other times, they are severe and life-threatening.

A special type of soft-tissue injury is a burn. Burns are classified by the depth of soft tissue that is burned (*superficial*, *partial-thickness*, and *full-thickness*), as well as by the cause of the burn (*thermal*, *chemical*, *electrical*, *radiation*).

As the first trained person to arrive at an emergency scene, you must be prepared to provide appropriate initial care to trauma or burn patients and recognize when advanced medical assistance is needed.

Expanded Chapter Content

Wounds and Abrasions

Superficial wounds and abrasions should be thoroughly irrigated with large volumes of clean water with or without soap until no foreign debris remains in the wound. Wounds heal better with less infection if they are covered with an antibiotic ointment or cream and a clean dressing is applied. Prior to the application of an antibiotic ointment on a patient, verify that the patient is not allergic to the medication.

Burns

Cool thermal burns with cold tap water as soon as possible; continue cooling at least until the pain is relieved. Cooling reduces pain, swelling, and depth of injury. It also speeds healing, possibly reducing the need for surgical excision and grafting of the burned area. Ice should not be applied directly to the burned skin because it can produce tissue ischemia. Burn blisters should be loosely covered with a sterile dressing. Do not break blisters—they improve healing and reduce pain.

Electrical Injuries

The severity of electrical injuries can vary from a slight tingling sensation to cardiopulmonary arrest and death. When electric current traverses the body, thermal burns may be present at entry and exit points along the internal pathway the current traveled across. Cardiopulmonary arrest is the primary cause of immediate death from electrocution. Exposure to low- or high-voltage current may cause cardiac arrhythmias. Respiratory arrest may result from the electric current causing injury to the brain or from paralysis of respiratory muscles.

Never place yourself in danger by touching an electrocuted patient while the power is on. If at home, turn the power off at its source—usually a fuse box. If the electrocution is due to downed power lines, call 9-1-1 immediately. All materials conduct electricity if the voltage is high enough. Do not enter the area around the patient or try to remove wires or other materials with any object, including a wooden one, until you are sure that the power has been turned off. It is necessary to activate EMS for any patient who has received an electric shock because the extent of the injury may not be apparent.

Chemical Burns

Brush powdered chemicals of the skin with a gloved hand or piece of cloth. Remove contaminated clothing from the patient, making sure not to contaminate yourself in the process. For exposure to an acid or alkali on the skin or in the eye, flush the affected area with copious amounts of water.

Sources

American Heart Association and the American National Red Cross (2010). Part 17: First aid: 2010 American Heart Association and American Red Cross Guidelines for First Aid. *Circulation* 122:S934-S946. http://circ.ahajournals.org/content/122/18_suppl_3/S394

Name: ______________________ Date: __________

Learning Activities

I. Multiple Choice

1. In the case of a minor burn, treat the injury initially by
   a. Rubbing the area with a cold stick of butter
   b. Applying ice directly over the burned area
   c. Covering the burn with a sterile dressing
   d. Holding the burned area under cold water until the pain is relieved

2. The most appropriate care to provide for a patient with a blistering burn includes
   a. Loosely covering the burn with a sterile dressing
   b. Breaking the blisters with a sterile needle
   c. Keeping the blisters uncovered, open to the air
   d. Wrapping the burn tightly with a sterile bandage

3. A person working with a strong cleaning solution accidentally splashes the liquid into her eyes. What would be your first action in treating this person?
   a. Call the poison control center.
   b. Flush her eyes with running water for 20 minutes.
   c. Have her close her eyes and massage the eyelids with your hands.
   d. Call 9-1-1.

4. A group of campers are sitting around a fire roasting marshmallows. One of the campers leans in too closely, and his sweatshirt catches fire. What is your first step in responding to this patient?
   a. Cool the burned area.
   b. Call 9-1-1.
   c. Perform an initial assessment.
   d. Put out the flames on his clothing.

5. In which situation involving a burn should you call 9-1-1 or go to the emergency department?
   a. A partial thickness scalding water burn to the feet of a 5-year-old child
   b. A partial thickness hot grease burn to the arm of a 50-year-old
   c. An electric burn to the lip of a 2-year-old child
   d. All of the above

6. The *Rule of Nines* is a guide used to
   a. Determine the depth of burn injuries
   b. Determine how much of the body is burned
   c. Describe the key steps in caring for burns
   d. Classify the various causes of burns

7. In caring for a patient of electrocution, you should
   a. Call 9-1-1 immediately
   b. Look for entry and exit burns on the skin
   c. Assess for heart problems
   d. All of the above

8. The care for a closed wound involves the application of
   a. Heat for 20 minutes at a time
   b. An ice pack for 20 minutes at a time
   c. Direct pressure
   d. Indirect pressure

9. What is the estimate of body surface burned in an adult patient who has partial thickness burns on the back, one arm, and one leg?
   a. 27%
   b. 36%
   c. 45%
   d. 54%

10. Which of the following types of open wounds has the greatest risk of developing an infection?
    a. Laceration
    b. Puncture
    c. Contusion
    d. Abrasion

11. You arrive at the scene of an emergency in which a 40-year-old man caught his hand in the blades of a snow blower. Four of his fingers are completely severed and the thumb is partially severed and hanging loosely. The type of injury to the thumb is called a(n)
    a. Crush injury
    b. Amputation
    c. Laceration
    d. Avulsion

12. You are providing care to a patient with a thermal burn injury. The patient has been removed from the source of the heat. What is the first step that an emergency medical responder should take to provide care for this patient?
    a. Cool the burned area
    b. Maintain the patient's body temperature
    c. Cover the burned area
    d. Minimize the occurrence of shock

13. You arrive on the scene where a building has collapsed. One of the construction workers is trapped in the debris. His left leg is caught between two large pieces of cement. This type of injury is called a(n)
    a. Amputation
    b. Crush injury
    c. Puncture wound
    d. Avulsion

14. Your patient is a 32-year-old man who has sustained an electrical burn to his right hand due to a malfunctioning toaster oven. What is the first step in the care of this patient?
    a. Inspect the hand for entry and exit wounds
    b. Perform a primary assessment
    c. Care for any life-threatening conditions
    d. Make sure the current is secured

15. You neighbor accidently spilled concentrated dry powdered weed killer on his bare hands and arms. He begins screaming in pain. When you go to his house, he is complaining of severe burning and itching of his skin. The skin is red and irritated. What is the first thing that you should do in this situation?
    a. Scrub the hands and arms vigorously with soap and water.
    b. Tell your neighbor to apply a topical antihistamine to his hands and arms.
    c. Brush the material off with a gloved hand or towel.
    d. Rinse the area with copious amounts of tap water.

II. Short Answer

1. A wound which does not break the skin is called a ____________wound.

2. Impaled objects should be removed only if the following two situations are present:

   1.

   2.

3. As an emergency medical responder, you are providing care for a patient whose arm was severed just above the wrist in a machining accident. While you apply a tourniquet to the patient's arm, another trained rescuer gathers the patient's amputated hand. List the steps that the trained rescuer should take to properly care for the amputated hand.

4. Fill in the chart with the three types of burns and the characteristics of each.

5. List the two "C" words that help an emergency medical responder remember the basic principles in caring for a patient with a burn.

   1.

   2.

6. What is meant by the term *critical burn*? List six situations that are characterized as critical burns.

7. Sometimes even the best care for a soft-tissue injury is not enough to prevent infection. What signs would you see if a wound is infected?

8. An object that passes through the body will have both an ____________ and ____________ wound.

III. True or False

_______ 1. Puncture wounds usually do not cause severe bleeding.

_______ 2. Cleaning a wound with hydrogen peroxide can speed up the healing process.

_______ 3. A good indicator of the severity of a burn is the amount of pain the patient is having.

_______ 4. Never apply ice or a cold pack directly to the site of a closed wound.

_______ 5. Apply an antibiotic ointment or cream to burn injuries to decrease the risk of infection.

_______ 6. Only second and third degree burns are included in the *Rule of Nines* guide.

_______ 7. Embedded objects should be removed immediately so pressure can be placed on the wound to stop bleeding.

_______ 8. The first thing to do when someone is in contact with a fallen power line is to keep a safe distance from the patient.

_______ 9. Full thickness burns are less likely to cause pain when compared to partial thickness burns.

_______ 10. The skin of a patient with a partial thickness burn is usually red and dry.

_______ 11. Carefully pull away any charred clothing that is sticking to the skin of a burn patient.

_______ 12. The main priority in the care of a major open wound is to control bleeding.

_______ 13. A major open wound should be thoroughly cleaned with soap and water.

_______ 14. In general, patients under the age of 5 and over the age of 60 have thinner skin and often burn more severely.

_______ 15. The largest organ of the body is the skin.

IV. Matching

	Column A	Column B
_____	1. The most common type of closed wound.	A. Abrasion
_____	2. Wound caused by friction or scraping.	B. Avulsion
_____	3. Torn earlobe.	C. Contusion
_____	4. The medical term for a cut.	D. Laceration
_____	5. Skinned knee.	E. Puncture
_____	6. Penetrating wound caused by a sharp, pointed object.	F. Crush injury
_____	7. Wound where tissue is partially torn away from the body.	
_____	8. Jagged wound caused by trauma.	
_____	9. Wound created by stepping on a nail.	
_____	10. Bruising of the skin.	
_____	11. Type of injury incurred from collapse of a structure.	

V. Scenarios

Scenario 1

Due to a power outage from a severe storm, a family decides to use a portable kerosene heater to stay warm. Despite warnings from the parents, a 6-year-old child touches the top of the heater with her hand. Screaming in pain, she runs to her mother who sees large blisters forming on the entire palm of her daughter's hand. (Questions 1–2 refer to Scenario 1.)

1. Based upon the information provided, this burn would be classified as a
   a. First-degree burn
   b. Superficial burn
   c. Partial thickness burn
   d. Third-degree burn

2. Describe the actions you would instruct the mother to take in caring for this burn. List them in the order of use.

Scenario 2

You hear what sounds like a gunshot in your apartment building. When you investigate, you find a middle-aged woman in the hallway of the floor below you screaming for help. She tells you that her husband was cleaning his gun when it accidently discharged. Her husband is lying of the floor with a gunshot wound through his right ankle. (Questions 1–3 refer to Scenario 2.)

1. This type of open wound would be classified as a ________________________.

2. Prior to administering care to this patient, what must the emergency medical responder ask the patient to do?

3. What care would you provide to this patient?

21 Injuries to the Chest, Abdomen, and Genitalia

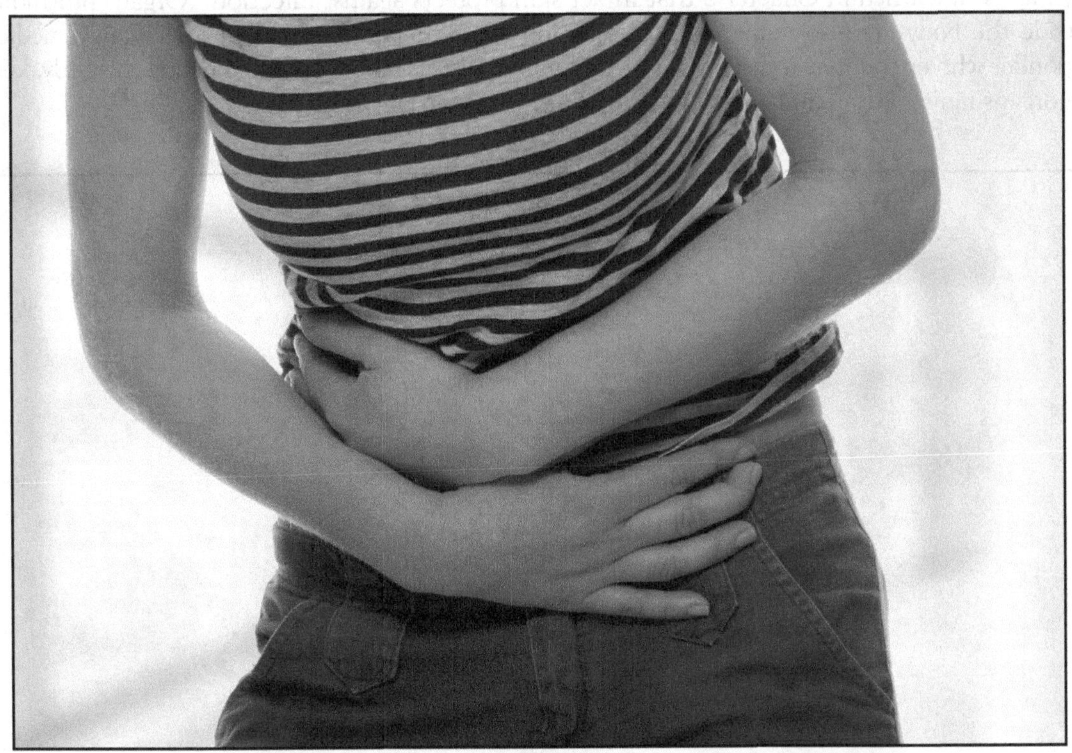

Chapter Significance

This chapter focuses on specific types of injuries to several body areas—the chest, abdomen and genitalia. Injuries to the chest can cause serious problems and death because the chest contains vital organs, the heart and lungs. An injury to the chest wall can occur as a result of broken ribs from a fall, or a wound as a result of a gunshot, stabbing, or an impaled object. These types of injuries allow air to be "sucked into" the chest cavity with each breath, collapsing the lung. This

CHECK ▪ CALL ▪ CARE

type of wound is called a *sucking chest wound* and needs immediate attention by an emergency medical responder.

Injuries to the abdomen and genitalia can also have serious consequences because these body regions are relatively unprotected by a bony covering. Any patient complaining of *acute* (sudden) abdominal pain should be evaluated by a physician; conditions can be mild such as an inflammation of the stomach and intestines to a life-threatening condition such as an *ectopic pregnancy*.

The proper care to provide for a patient with an *evisceration* is discussed. An emergency medical responder must remember that organs inside the body are moist and warm. When organs inside the body protrude on the outside of the body, they will dry out, become cold, and eventually die. You learned in Chapter 2 that intact skin protects against infection. Organs protruding outside the body are also vulnerable to infection. It is imperative that an emergency medical responder who encounters a patient whose abdominal organs are protruding outside the body, keep the organs moist, warm, and covered while awaiting the arrival of EMS.

Name: ______________________________ Date: __________

Learning Activities

I. Multiple Choice

1. Of the following materials, which one would be the best to use over a sucking chest wound?
   a. Gauze pad
   b. Elastic roller bandage
   c. Plastic bag
   d. Triangular bandage

2. To care for an open abdominal wound in which portions of the intestines are protruding outside the abdomen, an emergency medical responder should
   a. Attempt to push the intestines back in
   b. Cover the intestines loosely with dry, sterile dressings
   c. Apply moist clean dressings loosely over the intestines
   d. Carefully position the victim on his or her side, leaving the intestines uncovered

3. The main purpose of an occlusive dressing over an open chest wound is to
   a. Allow air to enter the wound
   b. Prevent air from entering the wound
   c. Control severe bleeding from the wound
   d. Prevent bacterial contamination of the wound

4. You are assessing a patient and notice a strange "whooshing" noise every time the patient takes a breath. You suspect the patient may have a
   a. Flail chest
   b. Pneumothorax
   c. Sucking chest wound
   d. Rib fracture

5. How should an emergency medical responder position a patient with a closed abdominal injury?
   a. On the side with arms flexed
   b. On the back with knees bent
   c. On the right side with the left leg raised
   d. Sitting up and leaning forward

6. A patient has fallen off a step ladder. During the fall, his chest hit the side of the ladder. You would suspect that the patient may be experiencing internal bleeding based on which of the following signs?
   a. The patient is coughing up blood.
   b. The patient's breathing is slow, 10 breaths per minute.
   c. The patient's pulse is bounding and fast, 100 beats per minute.
   d. The patient's skin is warm and flushed.

II. Short Answer

1. Pinpoint-sized red dots that appear on the head and neck following traumatic *asphyxia* are known as ______________________________.

2. The best type of splint to use for a patient with a chest injury is a(n) ______________________________splint.

3. Define the following medical conditions:

   Pneumothorax

   Hemothorax

   Subcutaneous emphysema

4. List five signs and symptoms of a chest injury.

   1.

   2.

   3.

   4.

   5.

5. How would you determine if someone has a *sucking chest wound?* What situations usually lead to this type of injury?

6. Define the medical term *evisceration.*

7. List all the steps an emergency medical responder would take in providing care to a patient with an *evisceration*.

III. True or False

_______ 1. The muscular partition that separates the thoracic cavity from the abdominal cavity is called the diaphragm.

_______ 2. Chest injuries are the second leading cause of trauma deaths each year in the United States.

_______ 3. Blunt force trauma to the abdomen can rupture the liver or spleen and cause the patient to experience hypovolemic shock.

_______ 4. Another word for asphyxia is *suffocation*.

_______ 5. The term *flail* chest refers to a simple broken rib.

22 Injuries to Muscles, Bone, and Joints

Expanded Chapter Content

- Fractures
- Types of Fractures
- Sprains and Strains

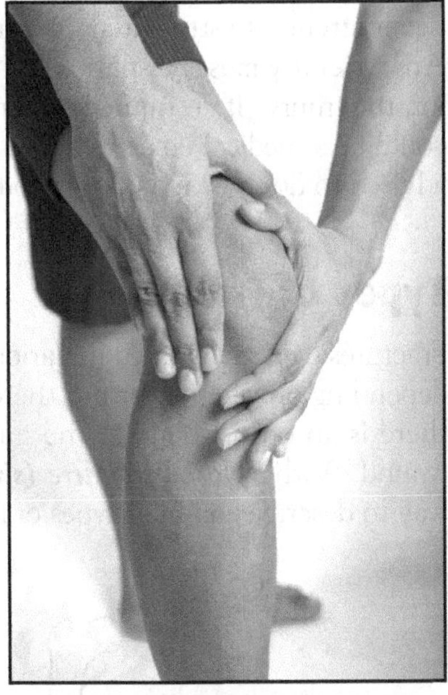

Chapter Significance

The musculoskeletal system consists of four major structures: muscles, tendons, bones, and ligaments. Traumatic injuries to these structures are becoming more common in adults, largely because people are enjoying a more active lifestyle and engaging regularly in recreational and sport activities. Musculoskeletal injuries are also common in the geriatric population due to different reasons. Elderly individuals suffer falls from poor vision, lack of muscle strength from inactivity, arthritic pain making walking difficult, problems with walking due to heart disease or diabetes (causing nerve damage in the feet and hands) and brittle, weak bones due to osteoporosis, especially in women. Musculoskeletal injuries can be serious and debilitating, particularly in the geriatric population, but they are rarely life-threatening.

CHECK ▪ CALL ▪ CARE

This chapter covers the four major types of musculoskeletal injuries: fractures, dislocations, sprains, and strains. You will learn how to rapidly identify these types of injuries and provide appropriate emergency care, including the immobilization of the injured body part through the application of a splint. In some cases, the type of injury may not be obvious (*fracture* versus *sprain*). When in doubt, assume that any injury to an extremity includes a bone fracture.

Fractures

A fracture is simply a broken bone. When a bone is broken, the surrounding soft tissue, nerves, and blood vessels can also suffer injury, resulting in bleeding, possible infection, and nerve damage. Assume that any injury to an extremity includes a bone fracture. Cover any open wounds with a dressing and never attempt to straighten an injured extremity. Splinting may reduce pain and prevent further injury. An extremity must be splinted in the position that it was found. The splint should be padded to cushion the injury. If an injured extremity is blue or extremely pale, activate EMS immediately because this could be a medical emergency. A patient with an injured lower extremity should not bear weight until advised to do so by a medical professional.

Types of Fractures

Fractures can be classified in various ways. The easiest method is to define the fracture as ***open*** or ***closed,*** depending on whether or not there is a break in the skin. With an ***open fracture (compound fracture),*** there is an open wound at the fracture site; in some cases, broken ends of bone protrude through the wound. With a ***closed fracture (simple fracture),*** the skin is not broken. Figure 22.1 illustrates another way to describe common types of fractures, that is, by the way they look.

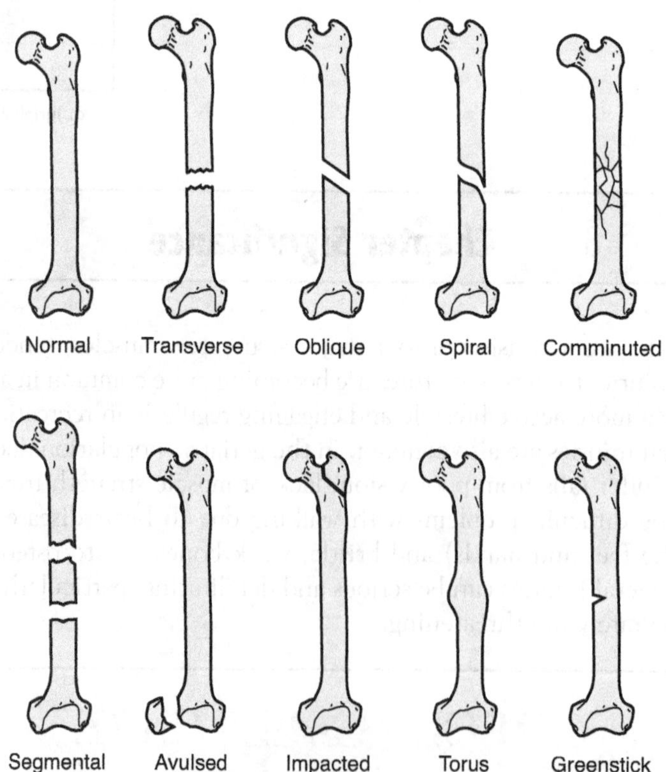

Figure 22.1
Common Types of Fractures

Sprains and Strains

The application of cold decreases bleeding, swelling, pain, and disability. Cooling is best accomplished with a plastic bag or damp cloth filled with a mixture of ice and water—this is preferable to ice alone. To prevent cold injury, limit the application to 20 minutes at a time and place a barrier between the cold container and the skin. The mnemonic *RICE* stands for rest, immobilization, cold, and elevate in the treatment of musculoskeletal injuries.

Sources

American Heart Association and the American National Red Cross (2010). Part 17: First aid: 2010 American Heart Association and American Red Cross Guidelines for First Aid. *Circulation* 122:S934-S946. http://circ.ahajournals.org/content/122/18_suppl_3/S394

Name: ______________________________ Date: ______________

Learning Activities

I. Multiple Choice

1. A fracture of what bone can cause serious bleeding and shock?
   a. Clavicle
   b. Humerus
   c. Femur
   d. Tibia

2. A sprain is an injury to the
   a. Bones
   b. Tendons
   c. Ligaments
   d. Joints

3. Musculoskeletal injuries are identified during the
   a. Primary assessment
   b. Scene size-up
   c. Physical examination
   d. Ongoing assessment

4. What is the length of time that ice or a cold pack should be kept on the site of a musculoskeletal injury?
   a. 20 minutes at a time
   b. 30 minutes at a time
   c. 40 minutes at a time
   d. Until pain and swelling are reduced

5. Securing an injured finger to an uninjured finger, in order to stabilize a suspected fracture, describes a/an __________________ splint.
   a. Anatomic
   b. Circumferential
   c. Rigid
   d. Soft

6. Which of the following conditions would alert an emergency medical responder to the possibility that the patient has suffered a serious musculoskeletal injury of the foot?
   a. The patient has a history of prior fractures.
   b. The foot is pale and feels cool to the touch.
   c. The patient exhibits decreased ankle motion.
   d. The patient has pain with weight-bearing.

7. A strain is caused by
   a. Injury to a ligament
   b. Overuse of weight bearing joints
   c. Overstretched muscles
   d. All of the above

8. You arrive at the scene of an emergency and complete your primary assessment of a patient. You notice what appears to be a bone protruding from an open and bleeding wound on the patient's lower leg. Which of the following actions should you take?
   a. Apply direct pressure immediately above the open wound.
   b. Apply a tourniquet to the leg above the wound to stop the bleeding.
   c. Raise the lower leg above the level of the heart.
   d. Pack the area around the wound with sterile gauze.

9. You are preparing to apply a splint to an open fracture of a patient's arm. The wound is oozing blood. What is the first action that you should take?
   a. Apply a dressing over the wound.
   b. Attempt to straighten the arm.
   c. Apply ice directly over the wound.
   d. Check the circulation below the level of the wound.

10. How can a dislocation best be described?
   a. The bone is broken or chipped.
   b. Two bones that are normally together become separated.
   c. The ligament at a joint is partially torn.
   d. A broken bone protrudes from the skin.

II. Short Answer

1. Identify seven signs and symptoms of musculoskeletal injuries.

   1.

   2.

   3.

   4.

   5.

   6.

   7.

2. General care for most musculoskeletal injuries follows the acronym *R.I.C.E.* What does each letter stand for?

   - R =
   - I =
   - C =
   - E =

3. Why are cold packs used initially on musculoskeletal injuries?

4. State the five purposes of immobilizing a serious musculoskeletal injury.

   1.

   2.

   3.

   4.

   5.

5. If you were to immobilize an injured wrist, the splint should extend from the _______________ to the _____________________.

6. An emergency medical responder remembers what to look for when assessing patients for musculoskeletal injuries by using the mnemonic _____________.

7. Name the six types of splints available to the emergency medical responder.

   1.

   2.

   3.

   4.

   5.

   6.

8. For an injury to the elbow, the bones above and below must be immobilized. Name those bones.

   Bone(s) above____
   Bone(s) below____

9. Define the term *cravat*.

10. Another name for the collarbone is the ______________________.

11. List the 11 rules for splinting.

    1.

    2.

    3.

    4.

    5.

    6.

    7.

    8.

    9.

    10.

    11.

III. True or False

_______ 1. Joints are stabilized by tendons which connect bone to bone.

_______ 2. The amount of swelling is usually a good indicator of the severity of a musculoskeletal injury.

_______ 3. Skeletal muscles are attached to bone by strong, cordlike tissues called tendons.

_______ 4. When caring for a sprain or a muscle contusion, apply cold first and heat later.

_______ 5. Squeezing and releasing the patient's fingernail is a method used to check circulation in the extremities.

_______ 6. When splinting the legs together, move the injured leg next to the uninjured leg.

_______ 7. A strain occurs when a joint is turned or twisted beyond its normal range of motion.

_______ 8. An injured joint should be straightened before splinting it.

IV. Scenarios

Scenario 1

You and your friend decide to take advantage of the beautiful weather by biking at a popular state park. While on one of the trails, you hear loud screams for help. You decide to follow the screams and find an elderly man lying on the ground, in the middle of a dirt path. He is bleeding severely from a wound on his left lower leg and a piece of a bone appears to be sticking through the skin. (Questions 1–5 refer to Scenario 1.)

1. What hazard at the scene must be addressed? How will the emergency medical responder ensure safety for the patient and self?

2. This man's leg fracture would be described as
   a. Closed
   b. Compound
   c. Simple
   d. Comminuted

3. What action should the emergency medical responder take before immobilizing the man's leg?
   a. Apply indirect pressure to control bleeding.
   b. Ask him to attempt to straighten his leg.
   c. Elevate the leg by supporting it with a rolled up sweatshirt.
   d. Pull on the leg until the bone drops into place.

4. What materials could the emergency medical responder use to improvise a rigid splint?

5. Is it necessary to activate EMS? Provide rationale for your answer.

Scenario 2

You are watching a group of young men playing basketball at a local YMCA. After several players jump into the air to block a shot, you notice one player come down and land on the foot of another player. The injured player falls to the floor, crying out in pain. His ankle immediately swells and turns purple. (Questions 1–3 refer to Scenario 2.)

1. To assess for circulation in the foot of the injured ankle, the emergency medical responder should
   a. Instruct the patient to stand and attempt to bear weight on the foot
   b. Ask the patient to gently move his foot and wiggle his toes
   c. Ask the patient about any areas of numbness or tingling
   d. Check the color of the nail beds of the patient's toes

2. To immobilize this patient's injury properly, the splint must stabilize the
   a. Ankle and knee
   b. Hip and ankle
   c. Foot and lower leg
   d. Entire leg

3. If a commercial splint is not available, what materials could the emergency medical responder use to fashion a soft splint?

Scenario 3

As an emergency medical responder, you are coaching your child's Little League baseball game. During the game, the pitcher is struck with a line drive to the forearm and falls to the ground. The child is crying and in pain, unable to move the limb. Swelling and deformity are present. The nearest hospital is only a few blocks away. (Questions 1 and 2 refer to Scenario 3.)

1. You rush over to assess the child and the child tells you that his parents/caregivers are not present at the game. How would you handle this situation? Can you provide care to the child? Provide a rationale for your answer.

2. You decide to treat the child by splinting the forearm. After the splint was applied, the child complains of numbness and tingling in the fingertips of the injured arm. What action should the emergency medical responder take?

Scenario 4

You are summoned to the scene of a collision between a bicyclist and skateboarder. Both were thrown to the cement pavement. Both were wearing helmets and other protective padding. Both are conscious but in pain. The skateboarder was struck on the outside of his leg by the bike. The leg is bent and his knee has an obvious deformity. The bicyclist was thrown over the bicycle handle bars, landing on her arms. She is bleeding from abrasions on both forearms. Her left wrist has an obvious deformity. (Questions 1–3 refer to Scenario 4.)

1. When you approach the scene as an emergency medical responder, what is the first thing to do?

2. From the information provided in the scenario, what other condition might these patients be suffering from besides musculoskeletal injuries?

3. You decide to splint the musculoskeletal injuries. What factors should be taken into consideration when choosing a splinting material?

23 Injuries to the Head, Neck, and Back

Expanded Chapter Content

- Traumatic Brain Injury

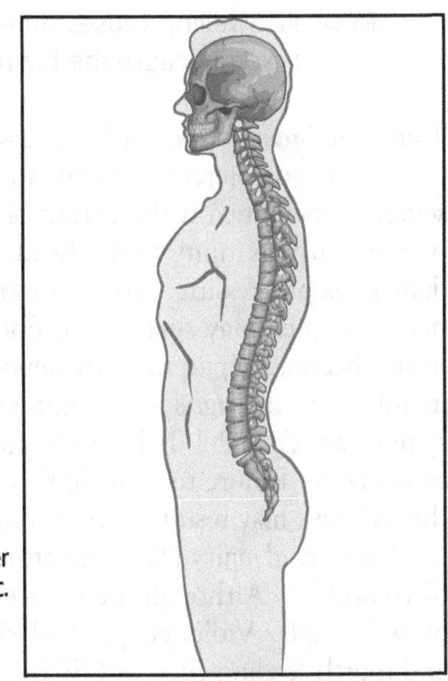

© Oguz Aral, 2009. Used under license from Shutterstock, Inc.

Chapter Significance

The brain is the most important organ in your body. It is the master organ, controlling all other body systems. Any injury to the brain will also impact other body systems such as the respiratory, cardiovascular, musculoskeletal, and integumentary systems. Injuries to the brain can be as mild as a concussion, or as serious as bleeding into the brain. The initial signs and symptoms that an individual experiences can be temporary, or can result in permanent disability. One of the most important priorities in caring for a patient with a head, neck, or spine injury is to prevent permanent damage to the brain and spinal cord; damage which is irreversible leading to *paralysis*.

As an emergency medical responder, one of your primary responsibilities is to assess the *mechanism of injury (MOI)* and consider whether the victim may have an injury to the head, neck, or spine. By identifying this type of injury, you can provide appropriate, timely care to limit additional damage to the brain and spinal cord.

CHECK • CALL • CARE

Traumatic Brain Injury

Actress Natasha Richardson died in 2009 from bleeding in her skull caused by a fall on a ski slope. Although the medical examiner ruled her death an accident, doctors said she might have survived had she received immediate treatment. Nearly 4 hours elapsed between her lethal fall and her admission to a hospital. Richardson suffered from an *epidural hematoma*, which causes bleeding between the skull and the brain's covering. Such bleeding is often caused by a skull fracture, and it can quickly produce a blood clot that puts pressure on the brain. That pressure can force the brain downward, pressing on the brain stem that controls breathing and other vital functions. Patients with such an injury often feel fine immediately after being hurt because symptoms from the bleeding may take time to emerge. To prevent coma or death, surgeons frequently cut off part of the skull to give the brain room to swell. Swelling causes more trauma to the brain which in turn, causes more swelling. This is a vicious cycle because the brain is located within the cranium, a closed space.

Traumatic brain injury (TBI) occurs when the head suddenly and violently hits an object, or when an object hits and pierces the skull and brain. The signs and symptoms of TBI can range from very mild to severe, depending on the extent of the injury. As an emergency medical responder, who is caring for a patient with an injury to the head, you must recognize when the patient's symptoms indicate that brain damage is progressing. You must keep in mind that a patient who has sustained an injury to the head, neck, or spine may seem to be fine initially; only later do signs and symptoms of brain or spinal cord injury become apparent. An important responsibility of an EMR is to educate the patient and family members on the signs and symptoms that would indicate worsening of the condition. If these signs and symptoms occur, 9-1-1 should be called or the patient transported immediately to a hospital for medical evaluation. Failure to provide this instruction to a patient, who later suffers from a disability caused by the injuries, may result in legal action being taken against you.

Spinal cord injury (SCI) affects primarily young adults, with most injuries occurring between the ages of 16 and 30. Although the most common cause remains motor vehicle crashes, the next leading cause of SCI is falls. Violence, particularly gunshot wounds, and recreational sporting activities, are the third and fourth leading causes of SCI.

The danger from SCI is paralysis, either from the neck down (*quadriplegia*), or from the waist down (*paraplegia*). A patient who is paralyzed has a permanent injury and faces lifelong confinement to a wheelchair. Many patients who are paralyzed die from respiratory complications.

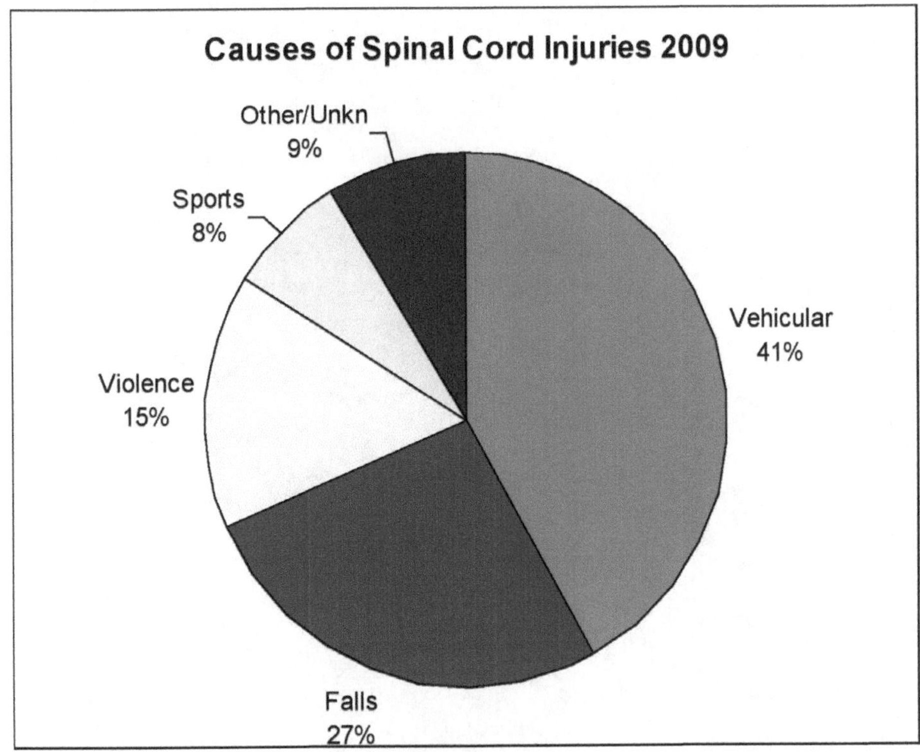

Figure 23.1

Source: Spinal Cord Injury Information Network—Publication of the National Spinal Cord Injury Statistical Center, Birmingham, Alabama. Spinal Cord Injury Facts & Figures at a Glance 2009.

Sources

American Heart Association and the American National Red Cross (2010). Part 17: First aid: 2010 American Heart Association and American Red Cross Guidelines for First Aid. *Circulation* 122:S934-S946. http://circ.ahajournals.org/content/122/18_suppl_3/S394

National Institute of Neurological Disorders and Stroke http://www.ninds.nih.gov/disorders/tbi/tbi.htm

Spinal Cord Injury Information Network – Publication of the National Spinal Cord Injury Statistical Center, Birmingham, Alabama. Spinal Cord Injury Facts & Figures at a Glance 2009. http://www.spinalcord.uab.edu/show.asp?durki=119513

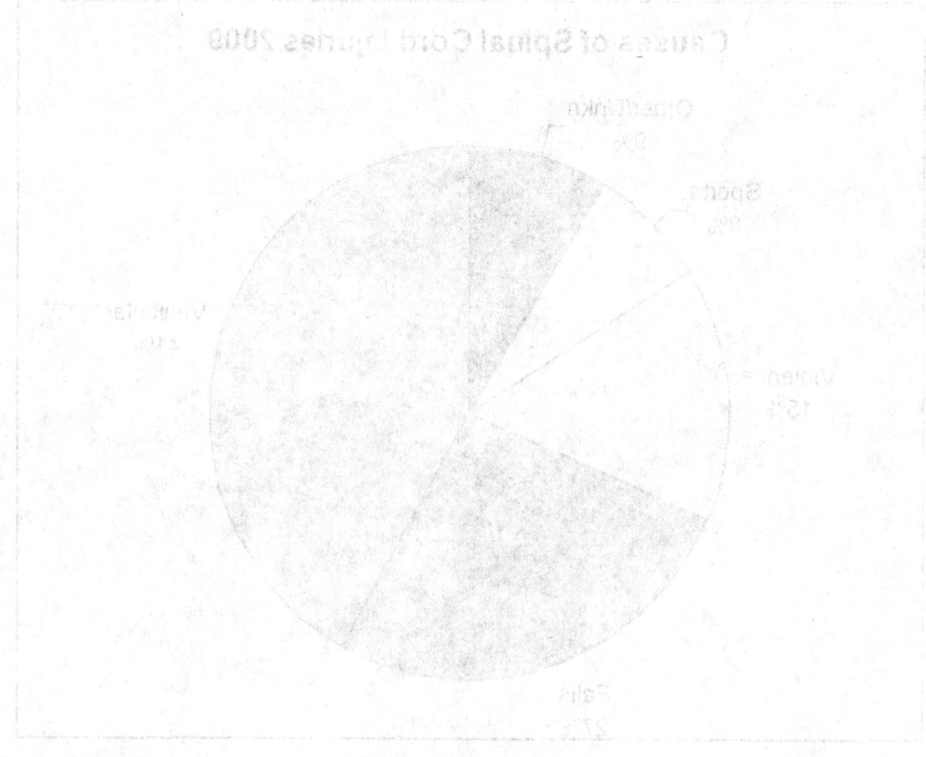

Name: ______________________________ Date: ____________

Learning Activities

I. Multiple Choice

1. Which of the following signs and symptoms may indicate an injury to the head, neck, or spine?
   a. Numbness and tingling in the extremities
   b. An inability to move a body part
   c. Severe and persistent headache
   d. All of the above

2. Most injuries to the head, neck, or spine are the result of
   a. Sport related accidents
   b. Motor vehicle accidents
   c. Falls within the home
   d. Violence

3. Which of the following mechanisms of injury (MOI) would alert the emergency medical responder that a serious head, neck, or spine injury may exist?
   a. A fall from a roof
   b. Being thrown from a car
   c. Being knocked off the bike and cracking the helmet
   d. All of above

4. As an emergency medical responder, you encounter a woman who has a small piece of glass embedded in her eye. She has no other injuries or problems. What is the first step to take to provide care for this patient?
   a. Place a sterile dressing around the object and control any bleeding around the eye.
   b. Try to stabilize the object with a bulky dressing, then apply a paper cup over the eye and secure it in place.
   c. After positioning the woman on her back, reassure her and tell her not to move the eye.
   d. Place a patch over the uninjured eye to prevent blinking or other eye movements that might increase eye damage.

5. A patient has suffered a laceration on the scalp. When you examine the patient, you feel a depression of the bone under the cut. What method would you use to control bleeding?
   a. Apply pressure directly on the wound.
   b. Apply pressure on the carotid artery.
   c. Apply indirect pressure around the wound.
   d. Place a sterile dressing over the laceration, but do not apply pressure.

6. An emergency medical responder can stop a nosebleed by instructing the person to
   a. Lie down and squeeze the nostrils
   b. Throw the head back and squeeze the nostrils
   c. Lean forward and pinch the nostrils
   d. Pack the bleeding nostril with gauze

7. While attempting to slam dunk a basketball, a front tooth of a basketball player became entangled in the net and was torn out. Bleeding from the mouth can best be controlled by
   a. Rinsing the player's mouth with cold water
   b. Placing a rolled sterile dressing in the tooth socket and have the player bite down gently
   c. Reinserting the tooth into the empty socket
   d. Applying an ice bag to the side of the mouth that was injured

8. Indirect pressure to control bleeding should be applied for which of the following situations?
   a. Injuries to the eye
   b. Fractured skull
   c. Embedded objects
   d. All of the above

9. You need to stabilize a patient's head and neck. Because the patient's head is turned sharply to the right, what is the first action that an emergency medical responder should take?
   a. Place one hand on the side of the patient's head to hold it in that position.
   b. Apply a cervical collar.
   c. Make sure that the patient's head is facing forward.
   d. Maintain the head in the position found.

10. You arrive at the scene of an emergency and suspect that the patient has an injury to her head and neck. The patient is lying on her back. How would you perform manual stabilization on this patient?
   a. Place your hands on both sides of the patient's head.
   b. Position her head in-line with the rest of her body.
   c. Apply a cervical collar
   d. Maintain the patient's airway.

II. Short Answer

1. Define the term *concussion*.

2. List six signs or symptoms of head and brain injuries.

   1.

   2.

   3.

   4.

   5.

   6.

3. Define the term *manual stabilization*.

4. How would you perform manual stabilization?

5. What is the care for a patient with a foreign body in the eye?

6. Describe the care you would give to a patient whose tooth was knocked out.

7. What modifications are necessary to take when maintaining an open airway on a victim with head, neck, or spinal injuries?

8. Under what conditions should an emergency medical responder remove a patient's helmet?

III. Scenarios

Scenario 1

You witness a car in front of you suddenly move out of the lane to pass a car close to a curve in the road. As the car passes, the driver over-corrects when merging back into the lane, goes off the road, and strikes a tree. When you arrive at the scene, the driver is slumped over the steering wheel and wearing a seat belt, with the airbag deployed. He is unconscious, cyanotic, and has a deep laceration on his forehead. (Questions 1–3 refer to Scenario 1.)

1. Identify the *mechanism of injury*.

2. What types of injuries would you suspect that this patient has?

3. Describe the specific actions that you would take to care for this patient.

Scenario 2

At work, you are summoned to assist another employee who has been injured in a 9-foot fall from a ladder. As you arrive, you see the person lying on the ground. She is trembling and moaning in pain. A bystander says that she landed on her back. The victim has not moved from this position. She says that she has tingling and numbness in her lower legs and feet and pain in her back. She also has a 2 inch laceration on the side of her head. (Questions 1–4 refer to Scenario 2.)

1. What is the first thing that you should do when arriving upon the scene?

2. Identify the *mechanism of injury* and the specific type of injury that you need to keep in mind when providing care.

3. What information in the scenario did you use to establish that this type of injury exists?

4. What specific actions will you take in providing care?

Scenario 3

You witness a bicyclist being struck by a car in a busy intersection. The bicyclist is thrown from the bike, striking her head (she was not wearing a helmet). The driver of the vehicle jumps out of his care and begins screaming "Oh, no." He appears agitated and is crying. As you approach, you see the bicyclist lying on her side, her arms and legs twitching. Blood is spurting from a deep laceration on her thigh onto the pavement. (Questions 1–4 refer to Scenario 3.)

1. As an emergency medical responder, what are the possible dangers as you stop to render help?

2. Based on the information provided in the scenario, what potential problems/injuries does this patient have?

3. What is the first action that an emergency medical responder should take in this situation?

4. Prioritize the steps that you would take in providing care for this woman.

Unit 7

Special Populations

24 Childbirth

Expanded Chapter Content/ARC Updates

- Four Stages of the Labor Process
- Use of a Bulb Syringe

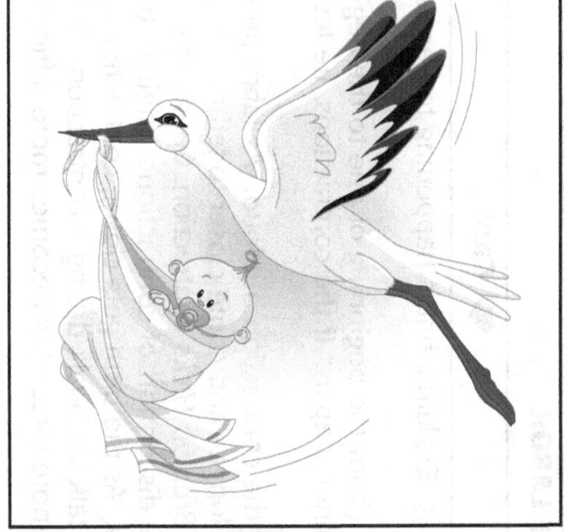

Chapter Significance

Although *pregnancy*, *labor*, and *delivery* are normal events that have taken place for thousands of years, as an emergency medical responder it is critical that you activate 9-1-1 if you find yourself in a situation where the birth of a baby is imminent. Even though the birth process is uneventful most of the time, there is always a possibility that something will go wrong; when events happen, they happen very quickly. It would be very difficult for you as an emergency medical responder to handle these unexpected situations. Even a patient with an uneventful pregnancy can develop unexpected problems during labor and the delivery of the baby. When you provide care to a woman who is in labor, you have to realize that you are actually providing care for two patients. Time is critical in ensuring the safety of both mother and baby. When problems arise during the delivery of the baby, the priority in providing care is always on the mother.

In this chapter, you will learn to recognize signs and symptoms which indicate that a pregnant woman is in labor, and the four stages of the labor process. Based on the information you have gathered, you will be able to estimate how much time there is before the birth occurs. You will learn how to make the mother more comfortable during the labor process and ways to expedite the baby's birth. The priorities in providing care to the mother immediately after delivery (*postpartum*) and the *neonate* (newborn) are emphasized.

CHECK ▪ CALL ▪ CARE

THE FOUR STAGES OF LABOR

Stages	What Happens	❤ Care
I. Dilation	• The woman's body prepares for birth. • Lasts from the first *contraction* until the cervix is fully *dilated* (10 centimeters) • *Bloody show* may be present • The *amniotic sac* (bag of waters) may be leaking or ruptured. • This is the longest stage; for first-time mothers, this stage takes 12–24 hours.	• Be calm and reassuring. Explain what is happening to her body. Remember, this is a normal process. • Time the contractions (from the beginning of one to the beginning of another) – "The contractions are 10 minutes apart." If the contractions are less than 3 minutes apart, the birth will be soon. • Count the duration of the contraction out loud. As labor progresses, the contractions become stronger, last longer, and come closer together. These changes do not occur in false labor, known as *Braxton Hicks* contraction. Counting out loud helps the woman to mentally deal with the discomfort of contractions. Initially, the contractions may only last about 30 seconds. As the birth gets closer, contractions last about 1 ½ minutes. At first, a woman can talk and walk during a contraction. As labor progresses and the contractions become more forceful, it becomes more difficult to walk and talk during a contraction. • Assist the woman to slow her breathing as there is a tendency to hyperventilate during contractions. To slow her breathing, ask her to breathe in through the mouth and out through the nose. Tell her to take a "cleansing breath" when the contraction ends. • Assist the woman to focus on an object. By doing this, she is not tensing up her muscles (including the uterus) during a contraction. By keeping the muscles of the uterus relaxed, the birth will progress faster. • Help the woman change her position. She can be up walking during contractions, as long as her "bag of waters" has not ruptured. To relieve pressure on her back, assist her to lie in a knee-chest position.
II. Expulsion	• *Crowning* occurs (the presenting part, usually the top of the head, is visible at the opening of the vagina). • Delivery of the baby	• When crowning occurs, the birth is imminent. • If the foot/feet or buttocks are visible at the vaginal opening, this is called a *breech birth* and presents risks to both mother and baby. • Most women feel a strong urge to bear down when crowning occurs. • Create a clean environment for the mother: place clean towels under her buttocks and legs and across her abdomen. Have a clean, warm blanket or towel to catch and wrap the baby in. Get a bulb syringe if it is available to use on the newborn. • Childbirth is a messy process – you will be exposed to blood and amniotic fluid so be sure to use BSI protection (gloves, mask, protective eyewear, and a disposable, waterproof gown).

Stages	What Happens	Care
		• Your responsibility when crowning occurs is to ensure that the head doesn't "pop out" quickly. The tissue between the anus and vaginal opening (*perineum*) is stretched very thin. If the head pops out quickly, the perineum can tear into the anus causing the baby to be exposed to feces and a potentially life-threatening infection. As the mother is pushing, place your hand lightly on the baby's head to allow it to come out slowly, thereby stretching the tissue gradually and avoiding a tear. • At no time should you instruct the mother to cross her legs to prevent the birth of the baby. Doing this deprives the baby of oxygen, leading to brain damage. • After the baby's head emerges, you must instruct the mother to stop pushing and begin panting like a dog. • Feel around the baby's neck to ensure that the umbilical cord is not wrapped around the neck, which can cause strangulation. If it is, try to gently slip it over the baby's head. • Next, suction mucus from the baby's nose and mouth with a bulb syringe (Figures 24.1 and 24.2). This is important because as the chest is squeezed through the birth canal, it causes the baby to take in a breath. If there is mucus in the nose and mouth, it will be aspirated into the lungs, causing pneumonia to develop. • After you suction the baby's nose and mouth, instruct the mother to push with the next contraction and gently guide the baby's body as it emerges from the birth canal. Do not pull the baby. • Have a towel or blanket in your arms, ready to catch the baby (it will be slippery). Towel dry the baby and then transfer the baby to a clean, warm blanket. • There are two priorities in your care of the newborn baby: 1. make sure the baby is breathing; and 2. keep the baby warm. If the baby is not breathing, flick the bottom of its feet or rub its back. If the baby does not begin breathing, give two ventilations. If the baby does not begin breathing, start artificial ventilations. Newborns lack the ability to regulate their body temperature, and they lose heat quickly. Keep the baby covered (especially the head), and place the baby on the mother's chest for warmth. • Obtain the first set of vital signs on the infant: breathing rate, heart rate, and skin color. (Continued)

Stages	What Happens	Care
III. Placenta Delivery	• The placenta is the organ that delivers oxygen and nutrients to the developing fetus through the umbilical cord. • The placenta begins to separate from the uterine wall with each contraction, and should be expelled from the vagina within 30 minutes.	• After the baby is delivered, the mother will continue to have contractions. Tell her that this is normal to expel the placenta. • Never pull on the umbilical cord to hasten the expulsion of the placenta. Doing this can cause the umbilical cord to be pulled away from the placenta, resulting in massive blood loss. • Save the placenta (place it in a plastic bag or wrap it in a towel) and send it to the hospital with the mother. The doctor will examine the placenta for abnormalities. • After the placenta has been expelled and the umbilical cord stops pulsating, tie the umbilical cord in two places: between the baby and the mother. Ties can be clean shoestrings or drawstrings on clothing. Don't cut the umbilical cord.
IV. Stabilization	• This is the recovery and stabilization of the mother. • This stage lasts about 1 hour. • Uterine contractions continue in order to stop bleeding.	• During pregnancy, the mother's blood volume increased by 50%; during the birth process, this excess blood volume is eliminated. Due to the sudden loss of fluid and blood, the woman enters a "shock-like" state following delivery. She is pale, shivering, cold, has an increased heart rate and respiratory rate, and low blood pressure. It takes about an hour for her body to stabilize. • Keep the mother warm; place warm blankets on top of her. • Give the mother plenty of fluids to drink. • Monitor her breathing rate, heart rate, and skin characteristics. • Clean the mother's genital area and legs of any blood. Place a sanitary pad between her legs. • Your most important responsibility is to prevent hemorrhage following childbirth. If you notice a lot of bright red bleeding between the mother's legs, you can control the bleeding in two ways: 1. ask the mother to nurse her baby. Sucking on the breasts causes the uterus to contract; when the uterus contracts, bleeding stops; 2. locate the uterus on the mother's abdomen (you will be able to feel a grapefruit size mass around the belly button which is the uterus) and gently massage it until it becomes firm.

Name: ____________________ Date: ____________

Learning Activities

I. Multiple Choice

1. Which of the following actions would be appropriate for you to take when the baby's head is crowning at the vaginal opening?
   a. Place your hand on the top of the head and maintain firm pressure against the head.
   b. Place your hand on the top of the baby's head and apply light pressure.
   c. Place the palm of your hand lightly against the baby's head.
   d. Do nothing and allow the head to emerge.

2. You are walking in the mall when suddenly a pregnant woman calls out, kneels on the floor, and clutches her abdomen. Of the following questions, which one would not be important in determining if the birth is imminent?
   a. "Is this your first baby?"
   b. "How often are the contractions coming?"
   c. "Do you feel an urge to push or bear down?"
   d. "Have you called your doctor?"

3. If the mother is having a breech birth, what part of the baby will you see first at the vaginal opening?
   a. Shoulder
   b. Buttocks
   c. Foot/feet
   d. Both b and c

4. Which of the following supplies should you have available to assist with the delivery of a baby?
   a. Umbilical cord clamps
   b. Sterile water
   c. Clean towels and blankets
   d. All of the above

5. After the baby is born, it is not crying and does not appear to be breathing. What is the most appropriate action for you to take?
   a. Give ventilations.
   b. Suction the baby's nose and mouth with the bulb syringe.
   c. Flick the soles of the baby's feet with your fingers.
   d. Administer oxygen if available and you are trained to do so.

6. An emergency medical responder can help a woman in labor cope with the pain and discomfort by instructing her to
   a. Focus on an object in the room during each contraction
   b. Assume a knee-chest position during contractions
   c. Breathe in and out quickly and shallowly during contractions
   d. Alternately tense and relax all the muscles in her body during a contraction

7. To help control persistent vaginal bleeding after a delivery, an emergency medical responder should
   a. Encourage the mother to nurse the baby
   b. Place ice packs over the lower abdomen
   c. Gently massage the area of the abdomen around the belly button
   d. Both a and c

8. The third stage of labor ends with the
   a. Delivery of the baby's head
   b. Dilation of the cervix to 10 centimeters
   c. Presenting part visible at the vaginal opening
   d. Delivery of the placenta

9. The placenta should be expelled within ____________ minutes after delivery of the baby.
   a. 10
   b. 15
   c. 30
   d. 60

10. You assess a pregnant woman who thinks she might be in labor. You suspect that she is having Braxton-Hicks contractions because
   a. The contractions do not get closer together
   b. The contractions do not get stronger in intensity
   c. The contractions do not increase in how long they last
   d. All of the above

11. Labor can best be described as
   a. The rapid development of the embryo into a fetus after implantation
   b. Rhythmic uterine contractions with cervical dilation leading to the birth of the baby
   c. Complete dilation of the cervix as the baby moves through the birth canal
   d. Birth of the baby with separation and delivery of the placenta

12. Which of the following leads you to suspect that the baby's birth is imminent?
   a. The woman reports no urge to push.
   b. Contractions are about 4 minutes apart.
   c. Contractions are about 2 minutes apart.
   d. The woman's abdomen is soft and relaxes.

II. Short Answer

1. Name the four stages of the labor process.

   1.

   2.

   3.

   4.

2. What specific techniques can an emergency medical responder use to help a mother allay her fears and relax during labor?

3. What does the medical term *crowning* mean?

4. In assisting with the delivery of the baby, what can you do to ensure the safety of the infant?

5. What are two immediate actions that an emergency medical responder should take after the newborn's head is delivered?

6. What does the mnemonic *APGAR* stand for? How often is the *APGAR* assessed following delivery of the baby?

   A =

   P =

   G =

   A =

   R =

III. Matching

Column A

_____ 1. Thick, pink, or light red discharge from the cervix.
_____ 2. The organ that provides oxygen and nutrients to the growing baby.
_____ 3. Also referred to as the "birth canal."
_____ 4. What a baby is referred to before the 8th week of pregnancy.
_____ 5. Movement of the fetus
_____ 6. Connects the baby to the placenta.
_____ 7. The organ that holds the developing baby.
_____ 8. Surrounds the developing baby and contains fluid.
_____ 9. Rhythmic tightening and relaxation of the uterus.
_____ 10. The process resulting in the birth of the baby.
_____ 11. The name given to a baby from week 8 until delivery.
_____ 12. Must dilate to 10 centimeters for the birth to take place.
_____ 13. The presenting part is visible at the vaginal opening.
_____ 14. The placenta peels away from the uterus prematurely.
_____ 15. The fertilized egg implants in the fallopian tube.
_____ 16. The baby's first bowel movement.
_____ 17. A baby born before 37 weeks.

Column B

A. Uterus
B. Amniotic sac
C. Abruptio placentae
D. Labor
E. Cervix
F. Contraction
G. Placenta
H. Premature
I. Umbilical cord
J. Vagina
K. Ectopic pregnancy
L. Fetus
M. Bloody show
N. Crowning
O. Embryo
P. Meconium
Q. Quickening

IV. Scenarios

Scenario 1
You find yourself in a situation in which a pregnant woman is very close to giving birth. Suddenly she looks to you with a startled look on her face. She tells you that she feels an urge to bear down and push. She looks very uncomfortable and is hyperventilating. (Questions 1–3 refer to Scenario 1.)

1. What personal protective equipment (PPE) would be important for the emergency medical responder to use when assiting with childbirth?

2. When you inspect the vaginal area, you notice that the baby's head is crowning. What should you do in this situation?

3. After delivery of the baby's head, what do you need to do before allowing the mother to push the rest of the baby's body out?

4. What are your two priorities in the care of the newborn?

Scenario 2
A mother has just given birth to a baby boy. He is blue, no activity or reflex, has a pulse rate of 98, is limp with no movement of his extremities, and is not breathing. (Questions 1–3 refer to Scenario 2.)

1. Based on your findings, what would be the baby's APGAR score?

2. If the baby is not breathing, what can you do to stimulate the baby to breathe?

3. What action must you take if the baby is still not breathing?

Scenario 3

A woman has just given birth to a very large baby after a long and difficult labor and delivery. When you assess the mother's vital signs, you note that her heart rate is high (125 beats per minute), her blood pressure is low (80/40), her respiratory rate is shallow and rapid (35 breaths per minute), her skin color is pale with cyanosis around her lips and nail beds. You examine the vaginal area and find large amounts of blood and clots draining from the vagina. (Questions 1–3 refer to Scenario 3.)

1. What conditions are happening in the mother *postpartum* (after delivery)?

2. What techniques can an emergency medical responder employ to slow down bleeding in the postpartum woman?

3. What care should be provided to the mother immediately after delivery of the baby?

Scenario 4

A pregnant woman is laboring in bed. Suddenly, she feels a gush of water and says she "feels something hanging down between my legs." When you examine the patient, you notice a loop of the umbilical cord protruding from the vaginal opening. (Questions 1 and 2 refer to Scenario 4.)

1. What is the first action that you should take in this situation?

2. If this situation is not resolved, what problems can this cause to the newborn?

Check-Call-Care: Use of a Bulb Syringe

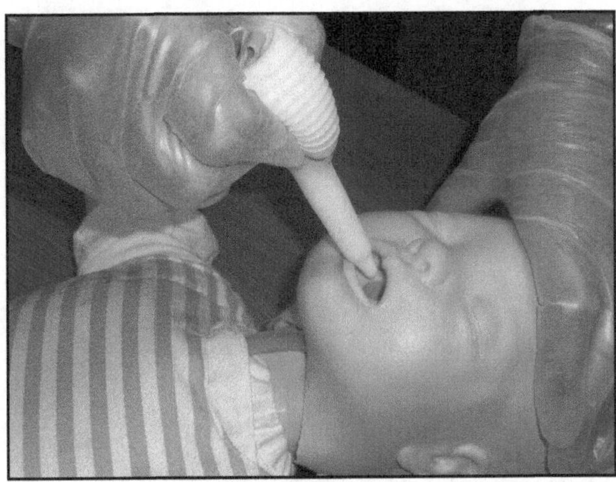

Figure 24.1
Squeeze the bulb syringe to activate the suction, before placing it in the baby's mouth. Suction the mouth then release the bulb syringe over a towel or gauze to expel the contents. Repeat as necessary to clear the mouth.

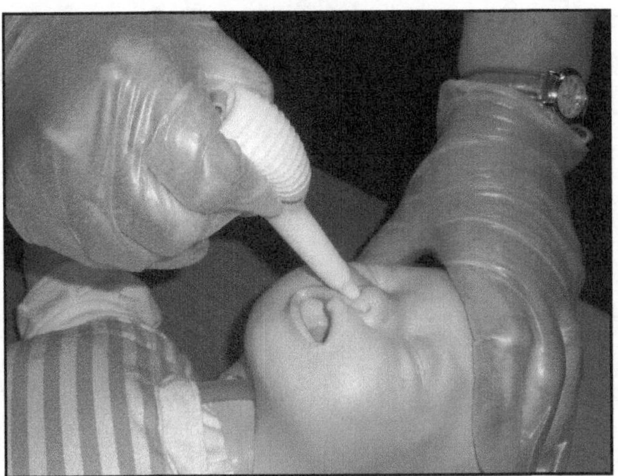

Figure 24.2
After suctioning the mouth, suction each nostril. Squeeze the bulb syringe to activate the suction, before inserting it into the nostril. After cleaning one nostril, squeeze the bulb syringe and insert it into the other nostril. Repeat as necessary to clear the nostrils of mucus.

25 Pediatrics

Expanded Chapter Content

- Developmental Characteristics
- Sudden Infant Death Syndrome (SIDS)
- Child Abuse

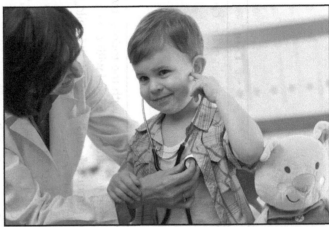

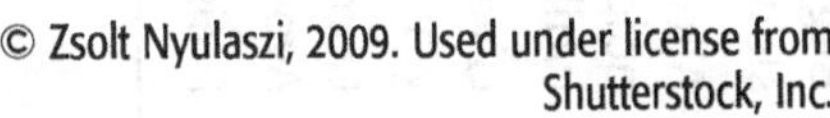

Chapter Significance

Up to this point, you have learned how to care for an ill or injured adult, one who understands your questions and can answer them appropriately. In this chapter, an emergency medical responder will learn how to modify that care to meet the developmental needs of ill or injured infants and children.

It is important to understand that children are not miniature adults. Children have limited cognitive abilities which impacts the way they understand words and questions posed to them. Their limited vocabulary makes it difficult for them to tell you about their fears, worries, or the pain they are experiencing. EMRs must often use their powers of observation to determine the *mechanism of injury* (MOI) and the *nature of the illness* when caring for a pediatric patient. In addition to cognitive differences, the emergency medical responder must also consider anatomical and physiological differences when providing care to this age group.

Although this chapter discusses developmental and structural differences common in *pediatric* patients (ages 0–12 years of age), a great deal of variation exists in the size and weight of children of the same age; this fact may require an EMR to also modify the care given to fit the size of the child. An EMR needs to remember that a sick child equals a sick family—one can't separate a child from his or her family. One of your responsibilities is to communicate effectively with the child and his parents/caregivers. Gaining the trust of the child and his parents/caregivers will allow the emergency medical responder to adequately assess and care for the child.

You will also need to be an advocate for children; if you suspect that any form of abuse is occurring, you have a moral and sometimes a legal obligation to report your suspicions.

Age	Developmental Characteristics	❤ Care
Infant 0–1 year	• Infants 0–6 months of age are easy to approach because they aren't afraid of you. • 6–12 months, "stranger anxiety" develops. Infants cling to their caregiver and are unwilling to allow you to examine/care for them.	• Allow the infant to remain in the caregiver's arms while you examine/care for him/her.
Toddler 1–3 years	• Toddlers are generally not cooperative. • They want to be autonomous and frequently say "No" to most requests. • Toddlers are very concerned about being separated from their parents/caregivers. • Toddlers have rituals and routines which allow them to maintain control over the situation. • Toddlers have trouble sitting still and dislike being restrained–they are always on the move.	• Establish rapport with the toddler by kneeling or sitting so that you are at eye level with the child. • Introduce yourself and ask the child his/her name, call the child by name. • Conduct an examination, or provide care, while the child is sitting in the parents/caregiver's lap or with the caregiver close by. • Begin a physical examination at the child's feet and work slowly to the head; talk to the child during your care. • Allow the child a sense of security by allowing him/her to hold a favorite toy or blanket during the examination or while providing care. • Give the child choices, if possible. For example, "Do you want this band-aid or that band-aid over the "boo boo." • Communicate by using simple words and short sentences. Avoid words that imply pain such as "cut." • Praise the child for his/her cooperation.

Age	Developmental Characteristics	❤ Care
Preschool 3–5 years	• Preschool children are very curious; they ask many questions, such as "Why are you doing that?" • Preschool children often have imaginary friends. They enjoy dressing up and playing make believe. • Sometimes, preschool children have difficulty figuring out what is real and what is imagined. For example, they are just as fearful of a needle going into their body, as they are of the needle being removed because they believe that "blood will run out of the hole." • They can tolerate brief periods of separation from their parents/caregivers. • They may be reluctant to allow you to examine them, or provide care, if they have been taught about "stranger danger." • Preschool children can feel guilty that they caused an injury to happen. For example, the child was told not to climb a fence. The child disobeyed the parent/caregiver, climbed the fence, fell, and broke his/her arm. • Preschool children are unable to adequately describe symptoms, and are unable to locate the source of pain. They speak in generalities such as, "My tummy hurts." When asked to point to the spot where it hurts, the child will rub the entire abdomen.	• Talk to the child to establish rapport. Introduce yourself and call the child by name. Get at eye level with the child during an examination or when providing care. • Tell the child what you see, and what you plan to do. • Use simple words and short sentences, such as "This will help your boo-boo." Avoid words that imply pain, such as "cut" or "take out." • Apply a band-aid over every "boo boo." • Allow the child to have a favorite toy or blanket for comfort and security. • Perform a physical examination beginning at the feet and work up to the head. • Allow the child to examine equipment prior to placing it on him/her. • Allow the child to place equipment (such as EKG patches) on a stuffed animal first. • Cover wounds so as not to upset the child. • Give the child choices, if possible. "Which band-aid would you like?"

Age	Developmental Characteristics	Care
School-age 6–12 years	• A school-age child is usually cooperative. • School-age children are fairly reliable historians regarding their illness or injury. They are able to tell you about symptoms they are having, the duration of the symptoms, and they are able to localize the source of pain. • They are naturally curious and want to participate in their care. • They often ask questions related to their illness or injury. • Secondary sex characteristics (puberty) begins to develop; they may experience anxiety during an examination of their body. • Like to collect objects.	• Talk to the child using simple terms, without "talking down" to him/her. • Get the child involved in his/her care. • Give the child choices, if possible. • Provide privacy and respect their modesty. • Inform them of any pain associated with a procedure before you do it. • Use distraction techniques such as a TV, IPod, or video games. • Use concrete terms and/or drawings to convey to the child where his/her injury is located. • May request to keep something related to his/her care or injury as a "souvenir." Honor this request, if possible.
Adolescent** 13–18 years **The American Red Cross treats children ages 12 and older as adults.	• Adolescents are more like adults than children. • They understand various diseases and the implications of disability associated with an injury. • Their developing bodies cause them to be modest. • They may not speak so freely in front of caregivers. • They are able to tell you about symptoms they are having, the duration of the symptoms, and are able to localize the source of pain.	• Protect the adolescent's modesty and provide privacy during a physical examination, or when providing care. • Examine the adolescent in private if he/she seems uncomfortable with the caregivers around. • Include the adolescent in the decision making process. • Interview the adolescent and parents/caregivers separately, if possible, to gain the most information.

Sudden Infant Death Syndrome (SIDS)

SIDS is the leading cause of death among infants aged 1–12 months, and is the third leading cause overall of infant *mortality* in the United States. Although the overall rate of SIDS in the United States has declined by more than 50% since 1990, rates for non-Hispanic black and American Indian/Alaskan Native infants remain disproportionately higher than the rest of the population. Each year in the United States, more than 4,500 infants die suddenly of no immediately, obvious cause. Preventing SIDS remains an important public health priority.

The cause of SIDS is still unknown; however, research has shown a strong correlation between the sleeping position of the infant and the incidence of SIDS. In 1992, the American Academy of Pediatrics (AAP) recommended that infants not be placed on their abdomens to sleep. A "Back to Sleep" campaign was initiated to educate parents, caregivers, day care center staff, and others to place an infant either on his or her back or side for sleep. Since this campaign began, the number of SIDS deaths has declined from more than 5,000 to less than 2,500 per year.

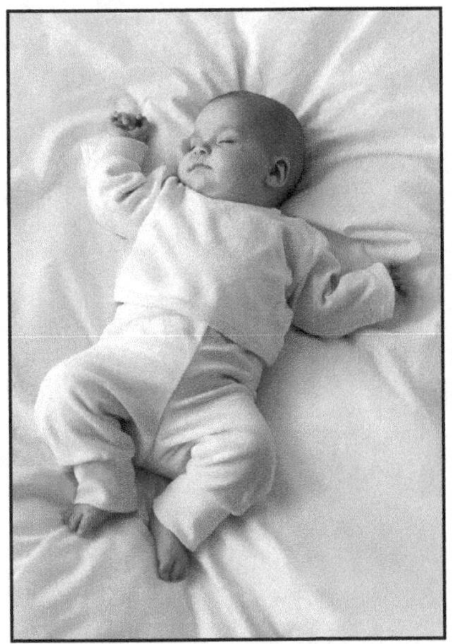

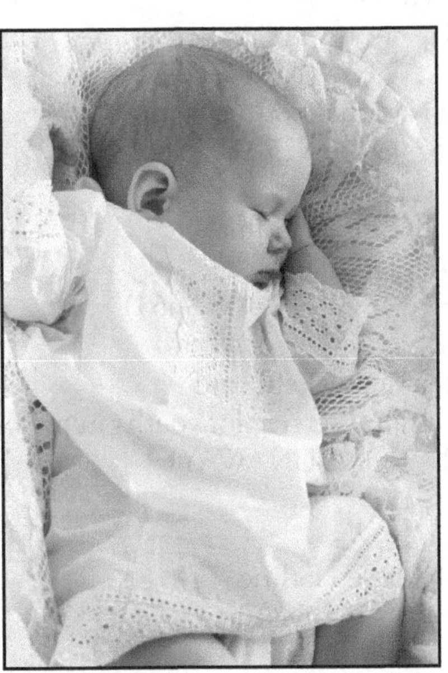

Child Abuse

A 31-year-old father was recently sentenced to life in prison for the death of his infant son. Before the infant boy was 1 month old, he was shaken violently and thrown to the ground by his father in a fit of rage. The father was irritated by the infant's fussy crying, a temper cut short by drugs and alcohol. The father initially gave various versions of what had happened to the infant, later admitting that he grabbed the baby and shook him before throwing him to the ground. The baby, who was on life support for several weeks, died as a result of a skull fracture, bleeding in the brain, and fractured ribs.

As an emergency medical responder, you may be faced with a situation in which the explanation given by a parent/caregiver of how their child's injury occurred is questionable. Your role in this situation is to first provide care for the child's injuries and then report your suspicions. In every state, certain individuals are legally required to report suspected abuse. As an emergency medical responder, it is your legal obligation to report your suspicions; in your chosen career, it may be your moral as well as your legal duty to report suspicions of child abuse. Remember that you must be an advocate for the child because an abused child typically does not confide in others about the abuse. If you suspect abuse, report it to your supervisor or the local child protective services department. Reporting may be done anonymously and without legal ramifications to you should your suspicions turn out to be unfounded.

Some individuals fail to report suspicions of child abuse because they see the physical actions of the parent as merely "disciplining" a child. Keep in mind that child abuse crosses all social, economic, and racial groups. When abusers are stereotyped as being solely from a lower socioeconomic background, many other abusers slip through the cracks because they don't fit the stereotypic profile.

Listed below are several child abuse hotlines and crisis-lines:

Childhelp USA®
National Child Abuse hotline
1-800-4-A-CHILD
24 hours a day

Child Abuse National hotline
1-800-252-2873, 1-800-25ABUSE

National Youth Crisis Hotline
National Youth Development
1-800-HIT-HOME (1-800-448-4663)

National Runaway Switchboard
(Hotline for referral service for youths in personal crisis)
800-786-2929 (800-RUNAWAY)

Stop It Now
Child Sexual Abuse Hotline
888-Prevent (888-773-8368)

Sources

http://www.cdc.gov/SIDS/

http://www.childwelfare.gov/responding/reporting

Moon, RY, Kotch, L, Aird, L. State child care regulations regarding infant sleep environment since the healthy child care America-back to sleep campaign. *Pediatrics*. 2006; 118; 73-83.

Newton, CJ. Mental Health Journal. April, 2001.

http://www.findcounseling.com/journal/child-abuse/child-abuse-laws.html

Vennemann, M., Bajanowski, T, Brinkman, B, et al. Sleep environment risk factors for sudden infant death syndrome: the German sudden infant death syndrome study. *Pediatrics*. 2009; 123; 1162-1170.

Name: ______________________________ Date: ______________

Learning Activities

I. Multiple Choice

1. Which of the following activities would help to develop rapport with an ill or injured child?
   a. Kneel at eye level.
   b. Call the child by name.
   c. Ask the child simple questions.
   d. All of the above would help.

2. An injured infant or toddler is most likely to be fearful of
   a. Car seats
   b. Separation from parents/caregivers
   c. Medical equipment
   d. Animals

3. Which of the following signs would indicate the presence of a partial airway obstruction in an infant or child?
   a. Retractions
   b. Cyanosis
   c. Inability to make sounds
   d. Loss of consciousness

4. The normal respiratory rate for infants and children is
   a. 8 to 10 breaths per minute
   b. 12 to 20 breaths per minute
   c. 20 to 35 breaths per minute
   d. 40 to 50 breaths per minute

5. As an emergency medical responder, you are caring for an infant with a possible broken arm and ribs. The parent's explanation for the infant's injuries seems questionable. In this situation, which of the following actions is a priority?
   a. Confront the parents regarding the infant's injuries.
   b. Treat the infant's injuries.
   c. Report your observations and suspicions to your supervisor.
   d. Notify local law enforcement.

6. Prolonged or excessively high fever in a child can result in
   a. Stroke
   b. Seizures
   c. Heart failure
   d. Breathing difficulty

7. You are dispatched to the scene of a motor vehicle accident and find a small child secured in an unbroken car seat. The child is conscious and crying. How should you examine this child for possible injuries?
   a. Leave the child in the car seat and examine the child there.
   b. Remove the child from the car seat and place him on a backboard.
   c. Remove the child from the car seat and lay him on the ground.
   d. Leave the child in the car seat and wait for EMS personnel to arrive.

8. Which of the following is the most appropriate way to cool a child down who has a high fever?
   a. Place the child in a tube of ice water.
   b. Sponge the child with cold tap water.
   c. Sponge the child with rubbing alcohol.
   d. Remove excess clothing or blankets.

9. When providing care to a child with autism, which of the following actions is most appropriate?
   a. Tell the child to look directly at you.
   b. Use verbal explanations of emotions.
   c. Expect the child to exhibit age-appropriate behaviors.
   d. Use touch to communicate with the child.

10. You are providing care to a 3-year-old boy with a respiratory problem. Which of the following should you identify as contributing to his increased risk for airway obstruction?
    a. Use of abdominal muscles for breathing
    b. Flatter shape of the nose
    c. Larger tongue within the pharynx
    d. Increased flexibility of the ribs

II. Short Answer

1. List three common developmental characteristics of infants, toddlers, preschool, and school-age children?

   Infant

   Toddler

   Preschooler

   School-age

2. How can an emergency medical responder communicate effectively with an ill or injured infant or child?

3. When providing care to infants and children, what modifications need to be taken during the assessment?

4. Define the medical condition *croup*.

5. Define the childhood disease *epiglottitis*.

6. List the care that would be provided to an infant or child who is experiencing respiratory distress.

7. Define the term *retraction*.

8. Unlike adults, children rarely suffer from a cardiac emergency. Instead, they suffer from a ____________________ __________________________ that develops into a cardiac emergency.

9. Define the term *febrile seizure*.

10. A high fever in an infant or young child is considered to be ______________ ° F or above.

11. Among children, the most common cause of shock is __________________ or ___________________________.

12. What is the leading cause of death in children?

13. What does the abbreviation *SIDS* stand for?

14. What is the cause of *SIDS*?

15. List four physical signs and symptoms of child abuse.

16. What is an emergency medical responder's responsibility if he/she suspects child abuse?

26 Geriatrics and Special Needs Patients

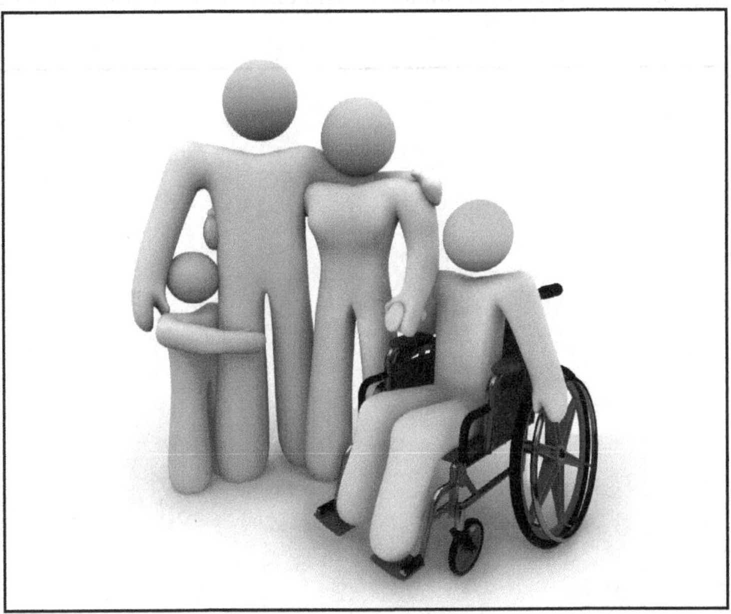

Chapter Significance

An emergency medical responder who is called to provide care to an elderly (*geriatric*) or special needs patient will need to modify the manner in which questions are asked and the way care is provided. An elderly patient who is afflicted with *dementia* or *Alzheimer's disease* will make it difficult for the emergency medical responder to gather information about an illness or injury, as in a *SAMPLE* history. As discussed in Chapter 3, it is very important to determine an individual's competence in these types of situations before care can be given. The emergency medical responder must also understand normal physiologic changes due to the aging process, especially changes in hearing and vision.

CHECK ▪ CALL ▪ CARE

Providing care to a special needs patient can pose many challenges for the emergency medical responder. An understanding of the pathophysiology of intellectual, physical, and chronic conditions allows the EMR to modify the manner in which information is gathered about the patient's illness or injury as well as how care is provided. Just as an emergency medical responder may question the competence of an elderly patient with dementia or Alzheimer's disease, the competence of a special needs patient may also need to be assessed prior to rendering care. It is important for an EMR to be able to communicate effectively with a geriatric or a special needs patient so that all understand the care to be given and the patient can provide consent.

Having a thorough understanding of the special needs that these patients have will allow for a more therapeutic approach to these individuals by the emergency medical responder.

Name: ______________________________ Date: ____________

Learning Activities

I. Multiple Choice

1. Older women are at an increased risk for fractured bones because
   a. Menopause causes a reduction in estrogen which keeps calcium in the bone
   b. The bones lose density as the woman ages
   c. The woman lacks a sufficient quantity of calcium in her diet
   d. All of the above

2. An emergency medical responder is called to the home of an elderly patient. Which of the following signs, if encountered, would alert the EMR to the possibility of elder abuse?
   a. The patient is taking blood thinners and has numerous bruises over both arms and legs.
   b. The patient has lost 5 pounds over the past 6 months.
   c. The patient was seen in the emergency room last year for a fall.
   d. The patient has poor hygiene and seems malnourished.

3. An inherited disease which causes mucus to become thick and sticky, obstructing the airways and the pancreatic ducts is
   a. Cystic fibrosis
   b. Multiple sclerosis
   c. Down syndrome
   d. Asperger's syndrome

4. Hospice care is appropriate to recommend for which of the following types of patients?
   a. Patients dying from heart disease only
   b. Patients dying from cancer
   c. Patients dying from emphysema
   d. Terminal patients who have 6 months or less to live.

5. Of the following behaviors, which one is often seen in a child with a diagnosis of autism?
   a. Repetitive behaviors such as playing the same game over and over
   b. Arguing and fighting with other children
   c. Enjoys being with parents instead of other children
   d. Talks to the family pet as if it were human

6. A group of genetic diseases causing progressive weakness and degeneration of muscles is known as
   a. Multiple sclerosis
   b. Cystic fibrosis
   c. Muscular dystrophy
   d. Cerebral palsy

7. Which of the following is most appropriate to remember when assessing and providing emergency care to an older adult?
   a. Clear, slow, calm explanations are important.
   b. Significant pressure is needed when giving ventilations.
   c. Dentures rarely interfere with maintaining an open airway.
   d. The older adult's skin requires less gentle handling because it toughens with aging.

8. Which situation most likely leads you to suspect elder abuse?
   a. A patient who attends a senior citizen center three times per week
   b. A patient with numerous old and new bruises on the arms and legs
   c. An elderly patient cared for by a live-in caretaker hired by the son
   d. An older female patient who suffered a hip fracture from a fall in the bathroom

9. A normal age-related change in an older adult is
   a. Diminished stiffening of blood vessels
   b. Enhanced sense of smell
   c. Widening of the aortic valve
   d. Reduced ability to hear high-pitched sounds

II. Short Answer

1. List five normal age-related changes in the geriatric patient.

   1.

   2.

   3.

   4.

   5.

2. When speaking to a geriatric patient, what modifications should the emergency medical responder make?

3. Define the medical word *dementia*.

4. What does the term *sundowning* mean?

5. State five risk factors for elder abuse.

    1.

    2.

    3.

    4.

    5.

6. List five signs that would alert an emergency medical responder to the possibility of elder abuse.

    1.

    2.

    3.

    4.

    5.

7. For a patient who is visually impaired, what modifications should an emergency medical responder make when approaching the patient?

8. Define *Asperger syndrome*.

Unit 8

EMS Operations

27 EMS Support and Operations

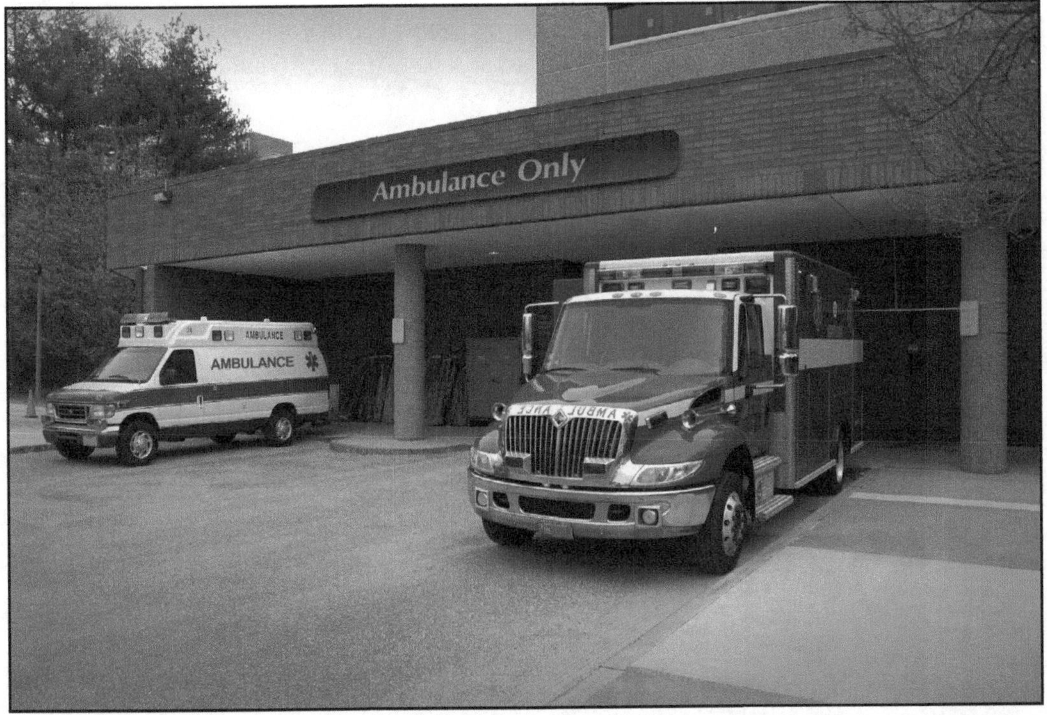

Chapter Significance

Because emergency medical responders provide a crucial link in the EMS system, they must be familiar with the operation of the EMS system and the roles that an emergency medical responder will assume during each phase of an EMS response. This chapter provides a brief overview of the typical phases of an EMS response to an emergency, from being prepared for a call through post run activities.

CHECK • CALL • CARE

Critically injured patients may need to be transported via air medical transport. When this becomes necessary, one role of an emergency medical responder may be to determine an appropriate landing zone and assist the helicopter to land safely.

Once a patient has been packaged and loaded into an ambulance, the EMR should be alert for road hazards which can impact the safe transport of the patient to the emergency room.

Name: ______________________________ Date: ____________

Learning Activities

I. Multiple Choice

1. Preparing the patient for transport to a medical facility is called
   a. Backboarding
   b. Dispatching
   c. Packaging
   d. Triage

2. You are called to the scene of a motor vehicle accident in which a truck has struck a utility pole. You notice the driver is conscious and seated behind the wheel, with a laceration on his forehead. An electrical wire is lying across the roof of the car. What is your first priority?
   a. Remove the driver from the truck.
   b. Stabilize the truck from moving.
   c. Remove the wire from the truck.
   d. Tell the driver not to get out of the truck.

3. The emergency medical responder is riding in an ambulance with a patient when the patient suffers a sudden cardiac arrest. Which of the following actions would be most appropriate in this situation?
   a. Ask the driver to hurry to the hospital so CPR can be initiated.
   b. Perform ventilations only since this can be done sitting next to the patient.
   c. Initiate CPR in the ambulance while taking safety precautions for yourself.
   d. Ask the driver to pull over while CPR is in progress.

4. You are performing a 360 degree assessment. This means that you are
   a. Ensuring that all equipment in the vehicle is secured
   b. Looking in all directions for possible dangers
   c. Identifying the need for lights and siren
   d. Checking the vehicle to make sure that it is in working order

5. In which of the following emergency situations is air transport least likely to be required?
   a. Passengers unrestrained in a vehicle that has rolled over
   b. A patient experiencing chest pain
   c. A patient who fell out of a third story window
   d. A building fire involving multiple patients with severe burns

II. Short Answer

1. Specially trained personnel who staff an EMS communication center 24 hours per day are known as ____________ ________________ ________________.

2. Air medical transport is requested for patients with what type of injuries?

28 Access and Extrication

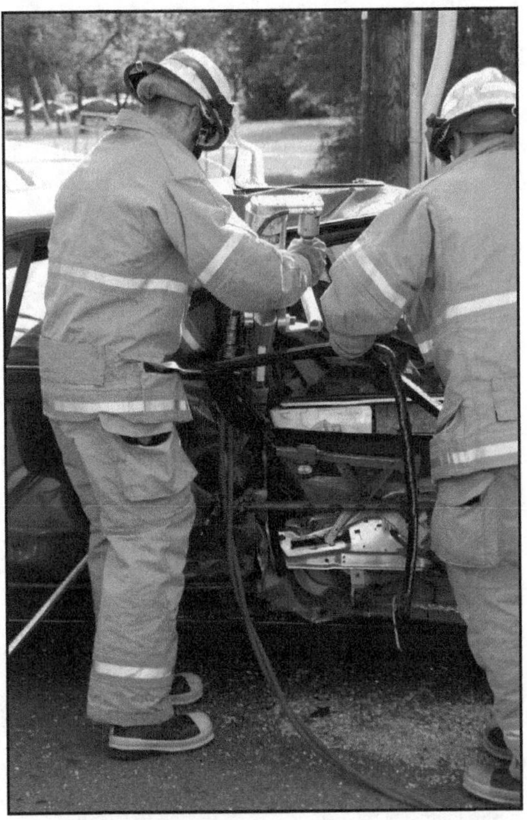

Chapter Significance

You learned in Chapter 5 that in most cases, the emergency medical responder will be able to render care where the patient is found. Moving a patient unnecessarily can cause further injury. However, there will be situations in which care cannot be provided to an ill or injured patient where the patient is located. Patients may be trapped inside crushed vehicles and must be removed either to provide care or because the scene is unsafe. The key words in this chapter are *access*, or

CHECK · CALL · CARE

reaching a patient trapped inside a motor vehicle or trapped in a dangerous situation for the purpose of *extrication*, or the safe and appropriate removal of the patient. Emergency medical responders must protect their safety by doing only what they have been trained to do, by using equipment that that they have been trained to use, and to wear appropriate clothing for the situation. Additionally, precautions must be taken to secure a scene or a vehicle before removing (extricating) the patient.

Name: ______________________________ Date: ______________

Learning Activities

I. Multiple Choice

1. Once you have gained access to a patient, the first action of the emergency medical responder should be to
   a. Treat the patient for shock
   b. Immobilize musculoskeletal injuries
   c. Remove the patient from the vehicle
   d. Perform a primary assessment

2. Which of the following actions would be most appropriate to take for a car that is upside down or lying on its side?
   a. Stabilize the car in the position it is in.
   b. Take the car apart.
   c. Leave the car alone.
   d. Turn the car in an upright position.

3. If an emergency medical responder encounters a patient lying across the seat, what is the first step he or she should take to remove the patient?
   a. Move the patient to the floor of the car.
   b. Move the patient's legs and body into alignment.
   c. Drag the patient head first from the car.
   d. Stabilize the patient's head, neck, and back before extrication.

4. The safe and appropriate removal of a patient trapped in a motor vehicle or in a dangerous situation is called
   a. Complex access
   b. Extrication
   c. Chocking
   d. Packaging

II. Short Answer

1. What is meant by the term *rule of thumb* in determining the danger zone area?

2. Which part of the patient's body is given the most important attention during the extrication process?

III. Scenarios

Scenario 1

You arrive at a scene in which a car has plunged down an embankment, landing on one side at the bottom. You can see at least two people in the car, one of whom appears to be conscious. Several bystanders have just arrived and are staring at the car. The doors of the vehicle don't appear to be damaged but you are unable to open them. (Questions 1–3 refer to Scenario 1.)

1. What are the possible dangers to you at the scene?

2. If one of the victims is conscious, what instructions would you give that person?

3. How can you ensure the safety of yourself and the bystanders in this situation?

Scenario 2

You arrive on the scene of an automobile collision involving one vehicle that has struck a guardrail head-on. The car is still running. The driver did not have his seat belt buckled and struck the steering wheel. He is seated behind the steering wheel complaining of chest and abdominal pain. The other passenger also was not wearing a seat belt. She is lying motionless, face down on the floor. You see blood around her body. She is unconscious and doesn't appear to be breathing. You are unsure whether she has a pulse. (Questions 1–5 refer to Scenario 2.)

1. What is the *mechanism of injury* in this scenario?

2. What precautions should the emergency medical responder take to ensure his or her safety?

3. Would you move either of these two victims? Provide a rationale for your answer.

4. If you do decide to move either or both of the victims, what precautions are necessary? What techniques would you use to move them out of the car?

5. What specific care would you provide to each victim?

29 Hazardous Materials Emergencies

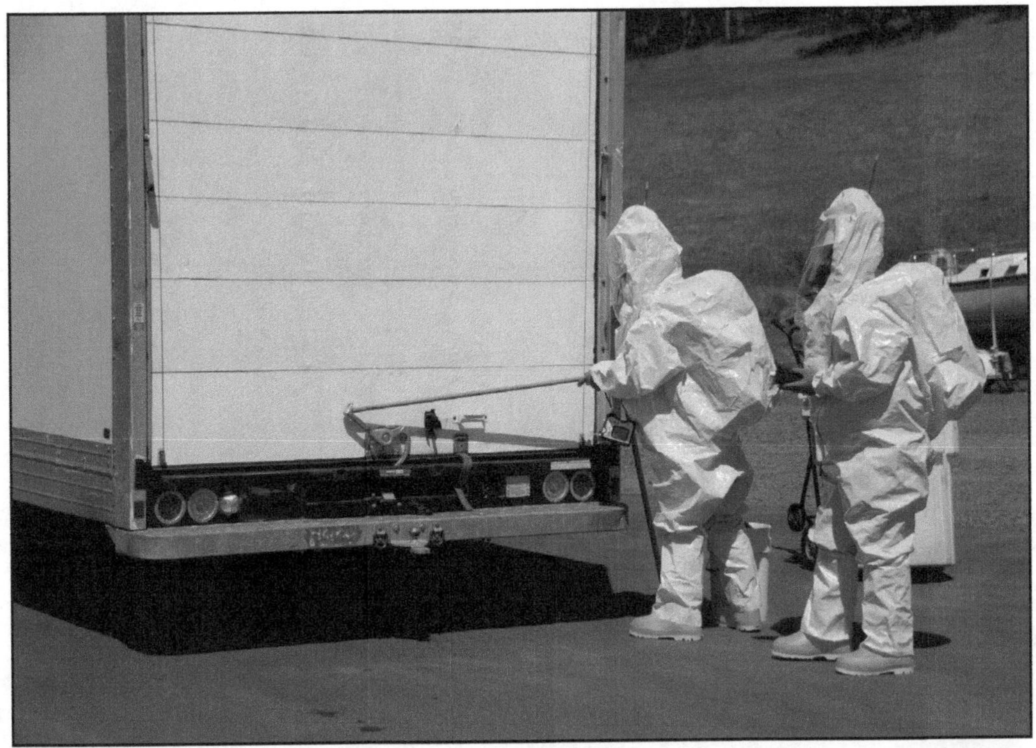

Chapter Significance

In every chapter, the safety of the emergency medical responder is stressed. Scene safety is especially critical when *hazardous materials (HAZMAT)* are present at the scene of an emergency. Hazardous materials can take many different forms: vapors, gases, liquids, or solids. Some hazardous materials have unusual or distinct odors; others are odorless. When an emergency medical responder enters the scene, he or she should look for the presence of signs (*placards*) which indi-

cate the presence of a hazardous material. The presence of a placard along with unusual liquids, vapors, gases, leaking containers, smoking or burning materials is indicative of an unsafe scene; the emergency medical responder should not enter the scene unless proper equipment is available and he or she has received special training in handling hazardous materials.

EMRs must be familiar with *Material Safety Data Sheets (MSDS)*, pages containing information on the physical properties and hazards of each substance. Another important resource where information related to hazardous materials and the appropriate care if an exposure occurs is the *Emergency Resource Guidebook*.

Name: ______________________________ Date: ______________

Learning Activities

I. Multiple Choice

1. In which section of the *Material Safety Data Sheet (MSDS)* would the emergency medical responder find information regarding a substance which is identified as being dangerous when exposed to other substances?
   a. Flammability
   b. Reactivity
   c. Toxicity
   d. Radioactivity

2. What types of activities occur in the "cold zone"?
   a. Patient rescue and treatment of any life-threatening conditions
   b. Complete decontamination of the patient and rescuer
   c. Support of the rescuers inside the exclusion zone
   d. Putting on a biohazard suit and a breathing apparatus

3. An emergency medical responder is exposed to radiation. The risk of exposure is determined by which of the following factors?
   a. Time of exposure, distance between the EMR and the source of radiation, and the amount of radioactive material the EMR has been exposed to
   b. Distance between the EMR and the source of radiation, the type of protective clothing worn, and the type of radioactive material
   c. Time of exposure, density of the protective clothing, and type of radioactive material
   d. Distance between the EMR and the source of radiation, the type of radioactive material, and the amount of radioactive material

4. The decontamination procedure that involves the use of soap and copious amounts of water is called
   a. Gross decontamination
   b. Dilution decontamination
   c. Neutralization decontamination
   d. Isolation decontamination

5. You have been selected to assist in a presentation about hazardous materials to a local group of emergency medical responders. As you prepare for this presentation, you research information about identifying and properly handling hazardous materials. Which of the following resources will you use to assist you in your research?
   a. *Material Safety Data Sheets (MSDS)*
   b. *The Emergency Response Guidebook*
   c. National Fire Protection Association
   d. The National Institute for Occupational Safety and Health (NIOSH)

6. You are approaching the scene of an emergency and notice a strange odor and a large cloud of gas in the area of the emergency. You would suspect the presence of which of the following?
   a. Explosion
   b. Hazardous materials
   c. Chocking
   d. Penetrating trauma

7. Which of the following would lead you to suspect that a hazardous material is involved?
   a. Mist
   b. Foul, acrid odor
   c. Broken glass bottles
   d. Downed utility wires

8. The best description of the term *HAZMAT* is
   a. The possible risk to health, safety, or property if the substance is not contained
   b. The probability that a substance is poisonous
   c. The degree to which a substance may ignite or catch fire
   d. The possibility of a reaction if a substance is exposed to another substance

II. Short Answer

1. What are *Material Safety Data Sheets (MSDS)*?

2. The hot zone is also called the ____________ ____________.

III. Scenario

You are the first emergency medical responder to arrive at a scene where a train carrying hazardous materials has derailed. (Questions 1 and 2 refer to this scenario.)

1. What clues would indicate the presence of hazardous materials?

2. Since the scene contains hazardous materials, what is the most important action that an emergency medical responder should take?

30 Incident Command Center and Multiple-Casualty Incidents

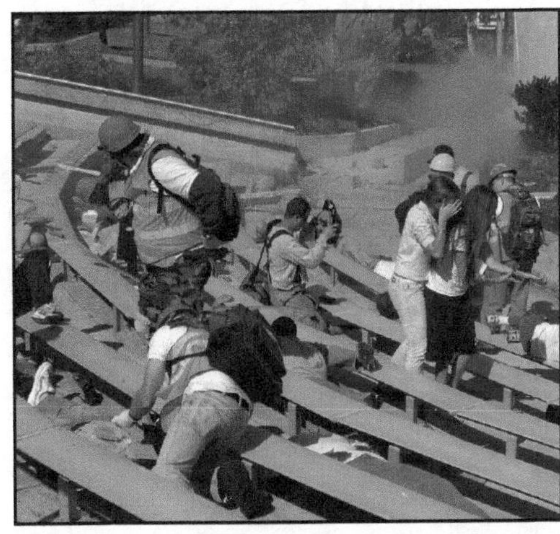

Chapter Significance

A *multiple casualty incident* (MCI), a situation involving two or more patients, can easily overwhelm the immediate resources of the EMS system. If an emergency medical responder encounters this situation, he or she must quickly assess each patient to determine whether the injuries sustained are life-threatening and require immediate care, or whether care can be delayed. This is the basis for the triage system, which prioritizes the level of care needed as immediate, delayed, ambulatory (walking wounded) or deceased.

In August 2011, a stage collapsed at the Indiana State Fair, killing five people and injuring 45 others. No one was performing at the time the stage collapsed. The opening act had just finished and the crowd was waiting for the main act to take the stage. The weather began worsening with heavy rain and strong winds. State police had been monitoring the radar weather reports and had made a decision to evacuate the grandstands; the plan wasn't carried out fast enough. The main

stage collapsed on a crowd of people after being blasted by wind gusts of 60–70 mph. Incidents, such as this, require numerous resources from surrounding communities and an organized system to manage the incident. This chapter provides an overview of the *Incident Command System (ICS)*, part of the *National Incident Management System (NIMS)*, which controls and directs the response for multiple casualty incidents.

Name: ______________________________ Date: __________

Learning Activities

I. Multiple Choice

1. An organized system of management used to control and direct resources at the scene of multiple casualty incidents or disasters is the
   a. Incident Command System (ICS)
   b. Emergency Control System
   c. Multiple Casualty System
   d. START System

2. The "big boss" who assumes ultimate responsibility in managing and directing the response at a multiple casualty incident (MCI) is the
   a. Incident Commander
   b. Logistics Section Officer
   c. Operations Section Officer
   d. Planning Section Officer

3. Classify the following patients into one of four categories, according to the START system.
   a. Immediate care
   b. Delayed care
   c. Ambulatory/walking wounded
   d. Dead/nonsalvageable

   _____ A patient who complains of a painful, swollen ankle.

   _____ An unconscious patient who does not breathe when the airway is opened.

   _____ A responsive adult patient who is bleeding profusely from a deep scalp laceration.

   _____ A patient complaining of severe back pain and is unable to walk.

   _____ An adult patient complaining of chest pain and breathing at a rate of 20–32 breaths per minute.

   _____ An unresponsive patient who has no pulse.

4. Emergency situations which involve multiple patients and may overwhelm the resources of a local EMS system are called
   a. Triage
   b. Incident Command System (ICS)
   c. Multiple casualty incidents (MCI)
   d. START

5. The so-called "walking wounded" would be identified by which triage marker in the *START* system?
   a. Black
   b. Green
   c. Red
   d. Yellow

6. Which of the following is used to manage an emergency situation and provide appropriate care?
   a. An incident command system
   b. The triage system
   c. The National Response Framework (NRF)
   d. The National Incident Management System (NIMS)

7. Which statement best describes the National Incident Management System (NIMS)?
   a. It coordinates the response to and recovery from disasters in the United States when those disasters overwhelm local and state resources.
   b. It is a comprehensive framework that outlines the structures for response activities for command and management.
   c. It is responsible for bringing together facilities, equipment, personnel, procedures, and communications within a single organizational structure.
   d. It is structured in five functional areas, including command, operations, planning, logistics, and finance/administration.

II. Short Answer

1. When using the *START* system, a patient showing no signs of life is left untreated. Why isn't CPR administered in this situation?

2. The process of sorting multiple patients according to the severity of their illnesses or injuries is called ____________________.

III. Scenarios

Scenario 1

A small commuter airplane carrying eight passengers and a crew of three has made a crash landing in a corn field. When you reach the scene, fire fighters and other rescue personnel are trying to extricate the passengers and crew from the mangled plane. (Questions 1–3 refer to Scenario 1.)

1. When you arrive on the scene, what is the first thing you should do?

2. What dangers exist for the rescuers and passengers?

3. Patients with which type of injuries should be treated immediately?

Scenario 2

You arrive at the scene of a train derailment. Two cars have been severely damaged and you are helping with the victims. The incident commander has assigned you to triage four patients, using the START system. One of the victims is standing, leaning against a tree. He says that he can walk. Another victim is lying on the ground moaning. You see blood around her body. The third victim is lying on the ground motionless, making no sound. When you check for his pulse, you cannot find it. The fourth victim is also lying on the ground, unconscious. She has a pulse but not breathing. When you open her airway, she begins to breathe. (Question 1 refers to Scenario 2.)

1. Using the START system, list each victim and the immediacy of the care that is needed.

31 Response to Disasters and Terrorism

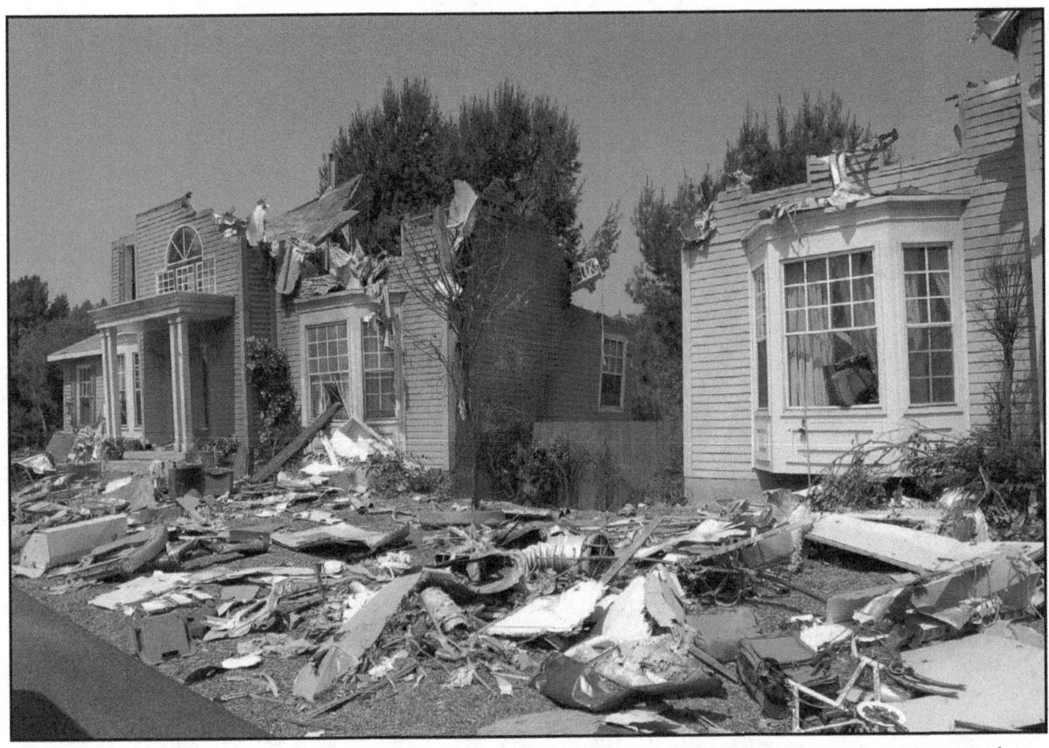

© Eniko Balogh, 2011. Used under license from Shutterstock, Inc.

Chapter Significance

An emergency medical responder may encounter a situation involving natural, human-caused, or biological disasters. When an act of *terrorism* involving *weapons of mass destruction (WMD)* occurs, the priority for the emergency medical responder is to ensure his/her personal safety as well as the safety of fellow rescuers and bystanders.

CHECK · CALL · CARE

Name: ______________________________ Date: ______________

Learning Activities

I. Multiple Choice

1. You are preparing to use the DuoDote antidote kit based on an understanding that the patient has been exposed to which of the following?
   a. Radiological/nuclear agent
   b. Nerve agent
   c. Biologic agent
   d. Explosive

2. Nerve agents are classified as to which type of weapons of mass destruction (WMD)?
   a. Biologic
   b. Chemical
   c. Radiologic/nuclear
   d. Explosive

II. Short Answer

1. What does the acronym *FEMA* stand for? What is the role of *FEMA* in disasters?

2. What is the FBI definition of *terrorism*?

3. Weapons of mass destruction (*WMDs*) are often classified by the acronyms *CBRNE* and *B NICE*. What does each letter stand for in these acronyms?

CBRNE	**B NICE**
C:	B:
B:	N:
R:	I:
N:	C:
E:	E:

4. Define the terms *mortality* and *morbidity*.

32 Special Operations

Chapter Significance

In this chapter, methods of rescuing patients from perilous and treacherous situations are discussed. Examples of such situations include water rescues, ice rescues, hazardous terrain, cave-ins, crime scenes, and fires. Since the rescue of patients caught in these situations is particularly dangerous, the emergency medical responder should be properly trained and have access to specialized equipment prior to proceeding with any rescue attempts. The emergency medical responder must keep in mind that special operation units are often necessary to assist in these unique rescue efforts.

CHECK ▪ CALL ▪ CARE

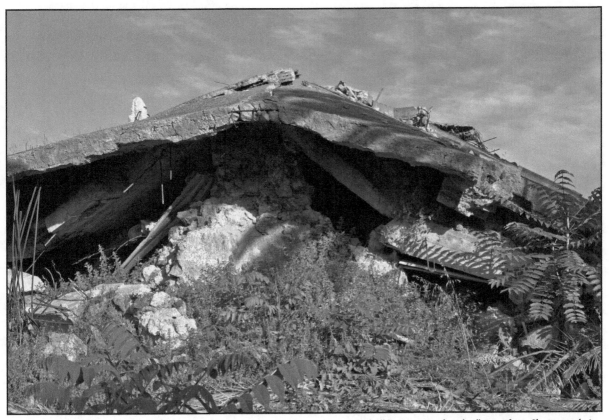

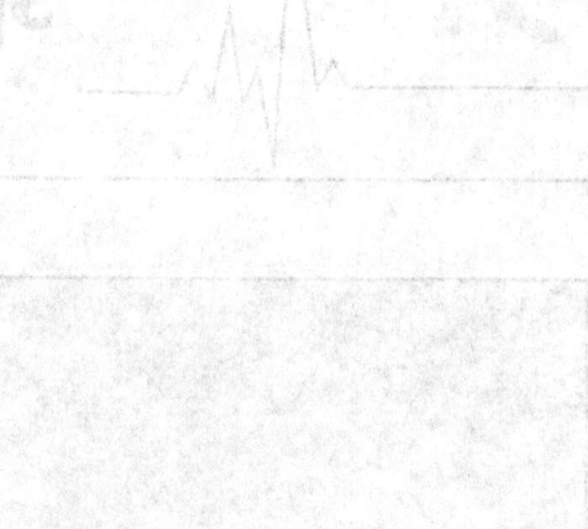

Name: ______________________________ Date: ______________

Learning Activities

I. Multiple Choice

1. A person is trapped in a farm silo. What type of situation is this?
   a. Hazardous terrain
   b. Cave-in
   c. Confined space
   d. High-angle situation

II. Short Answer

1. Define the following terms:
   a. Distressed swimmer

   b. Drowning victim—active

   c. Drowning victim—passive

2. How can you assist a person who has fallen through thin ice?

3. What is a *litter*?

4. State the reasons why a fall into a silo is life threatening.

5. List five basic guidelines that one should follow in the event of a fire if the person lacks either proper equipment or training.

III. Scenarios

Scenario 1

In August 2011, at 5:30 am, a pickup truck attempted to merge on 1-475N from Dussell Drive and collided with a semi. The pickup truck was disabled in the roadway while the semi pulled off onto the shoulder of the bridge overpass. Two women stopped to offer assistance. The first woman drove ahead of the pickup truck, parked her car and began running along the roadway to offer assistance. The second woman, who was driving a tanker truck, parked the vehicle north of the accident and was running back along the roadway to help. In the meantime, the driver of another semi, who didn't notice the disabled pickup truck in the middle of the road, and a man riding a motorcycle, both slammed into the pickup truck. Three people were killed: the driver of the pickup truck, the driver of the motorcycle, and the first woman who stopped to help–she was struck by the vehicles in the second crash. The second woman jumped off the viaduct to avoid being struck by careening wreckage and was in critical condition. (Questions 1–4 refer to Scenario 1.)

1. Looking at the events that transpired in this deadly crash, what could have been done differently to avoid the same consequences?

2. What are some possible dangers in this scene?

3. What would you do if you saw a placard on the side of one of the semi-trailers involved in the collisions?

   What would that indicate to you?

4. You proceed down the embankment of the overpass to render care to the woman who jumped. What type of injuries might this woman have sustained?

Scenario 2

You and another rescuer are searching for a missing hiker. You find the victim at the bottom of a ravine where he fell and injured one leg. He is in severe pain and unable to walk. The sides of the ravine are steep. A rapidly approaching storm threatens to flood the ravine. (Questions 1 – 3 refer to Scenario 2.)

1. How will you reach the hiker in the ravine?

2. Since the hiker has injured his leg and unable to walk, how will you pull him out of the ravine?

3. You decide to splint the hiker's leg. What materials can be used?

Scenario 3
A 36-year-old Green Beret died near Fort Bragg, North Carolina, trying to save his two daughters from a house fire. The parents woke up and escaped the blaze by jumping out of the second story of the home. The father wrapped himself in a blanket and rushed back into the house to rescue his two young daughters who were trapped in a second floor bedroom. The girls and the father perished in the blaze. (Questions 1–3 refer to Scenario 3.)

1. Should the man have re-entered the burning home? Provide a rationale for your answer.

2. Without further details as to where the blaze started or the layout of the home, what actions could the parents have taken prior to jumping out the window?

3. If the father had been able to rescue the two girls, what would be your immediate care for the girls?

A Appendix

FIRST AID FACTS OR FICTION: TEST YOUR KNOWLEDGE

Do you feel prepared to handle the most common types of injuries or illnesses that might occur in your home or community? Put your knowledge of First Aid to the test.

Question	Pre-Test	Post-Test
1. A person suffering from a nose bleed should be positioned with the head back and nose pinched.	T F Do Not Know	T F Do Not Know
2. If someone faints, splash cold water on his/her face.	T F Do Not Know	T F Do Not Know
3. To treat frostbite, rub or massage the affected area to re-warm it.	T F Do Not Know	T F Do Not Know
4. If a person begins having a seizure, place something in the mouth so the tongue is not swallowed.	T F Do Not Know	T F Do Not Know
5. Give glucose (sugar) to a patient suspected of having a hypoglycemic reaction.	T F Do Not Know	T F Do Not Know
6. If a person who is choking is coughing forcefully, give abdominal thrusts.	T F Do Not Know	T F Do Not Know
7. Never place butter on a burn.	T F Do Not Know	T F Do Not Know
8. When performing CPR on an adult, give 30 compressions and 2 ventilations.	T F Do Not Know	T F Do Not Know
9. If a child knocks out one of his/her teeth, place the tooth in a cup of milk.	T F Do Not Know	T F Do Not Know
10. Immediately apply heat to any musculoskeletal injury to reduce swelling.	T F Do Not Know	T F Do Not Know
11. Remove a stinger from a bee bite wound by using tweezers.	T F Do Not Know	T F Do Not Know
12. The first step in treating a burn is to run cool water over the affected area.	T F Do Not Know	T F Do Not Know
13. An unconscious, non-breathing patient requires artificial ventilations	T F Do Not Know	T F Do Not Know
14. If someone swallows a poisonous substance, immediately induce vomiting.	T F Do Not Know	T F Do Not Know
15. Remove an embedded object from a wound so that bleeding can be controlled.	T F Do Not Know	T F Do Not Know
16. The most effective way to control severe bleeding from an arm or leg wound is to raise the arm/leg above the level of the heart.	T F Do Not Know	T F Do Not Know
17. The acronym "AED" stands for ambulance emergency device.	T F Do Not Know	T F Do Not Know
18. The normal resting heart rate for a child is faster than an adult's heart rate.	T F Do Not Know	T F Do Not Know
19. The best position for an unconscious breathing patient is on his side.	T F Do Not Know	T F Do Not Know
20. Apply ice to a snakebite wound.	T F Do Not Know	T F Do Not Know

Question	Pre-Test	Post-Test
21. Most communities use 9-1-1 as their emergency telephone number	T F Do Not Know	T F Do Not Know
22.Chest discomfort is one of the most frequent signals of a heart attack	T F Do Not Know	T F Do Not Know
23. A person's airway can be opened by tilting the head back and lifting the chin.	T F Do Not Know	T F Do Not Know
24. A splint is used to stabilize or reduce movement of a broken bone.	T F Do Not Know	T F Do Not Know
25. Most injured individuals require a complete physical examination.	T F Do Not Know	T F Do Not Know
26. Activated charcoal is a substance that a poison control center may ask you to administer to a person who ingested a poison.	T F Do Not Know	T F Do Not Know
27. Salt tablets should be given to a person suffering from a heat emergency.	T F Do Not Know	T F Do Not Know
28. Hypothermia (low body temperature) occurs only in subfreezing temperatures.	T F Do Not Know	T F Do Not Know
29. Extremely hot skin indicates heat exhaustion.	T F Do Not Know	T F Do Not Know
30. An AED cannot be used on an infant or child.	T F Do Not Know	T F Do Not Know

Personal Health Inventory

Complete the **Personal Health Inventory** below. Are there areas in which you can make changes to improve your health?

PERSONAL HEALTH INVENTORY*		
Heredity: A member of my immediate family has been diagnosed with	**YES**	**NO**
1. Heart disease		
2. Glaucoma		
3. High-Blood Pressure		
4. Diabetes		
5. Asthma		
6. Depression		
7. Alcoholism		
8. Cancer		
9. Schizophrenia		
10. Obesity		
Total		

Mental Health	**Usually (always)**	**Sometimes**	**Rarely**
11. I am able to cry when necessary.			
12. I can adequately express feelings such as love, fear, and anger.			
13. I have a support system of friends and relatives with whom I can discuss problems.			
14. I control anxiety so that it does not interfere with my activities at school or at home.			
15. I am able to deal with stress so that I do not experience headaches or an upset stomach.			
16. I engage in hobbies that help get me to relax.			
Nutrition			
17. I eat a well-balanced diet containing meat, milk, fruits and vegetables, bread and cereals.			
18. I avoid foods high in simple sugars (e.g., cake, donuts, or cookies).			
19. I avoid using a salt shaker at the table.			
20. I avoid eating a lot of foods that are high in fat.			
21. I eat breakfast on most days.			
22. I avoid snacking between meals.			
Physical Fitness			
23. I engage in vigorous exercise at least three times per week (e.g., running, swimming, biking, tennis).			
24. I include exercises that build muscle strength and endurance in my exercise program.			
25. Prior to exercising, I perform stretching exercises.			

Physical Fitness	Usually (always)	Sometimes	Rarely
26. I make sure to warm up before and cool down after exercising.			
27. I engage in recreational and leisure activities that I can continue throughout my life.			
28. I maintain a healthy level of body fat.			
29. I get at least 7 to 9 hours of sleep each night.			
Personal Health Care			
30. I brush and floss my teeth at least once daily.			
31. I always apply sunscreen or sunblock, with an SPF of at least 15 for prolonged sun exposure.			
32. I have my teeth professionally cleaned twice a year.			
33. I have a physical examination performed every 2 years by my family doctor.			
34. When under medical treatment, I follow my doctor's instructions regarding taking prescribed medications and/or limiting my physical activities.			
35. I avoid the use of nonprescription drugs, and limit alcohol use and/or tobacco use.			
36. I have my blood pressure checked at least once a year.			
37. I am aware of the seven warning signs of cancer.			
38. I practice monthly self-examinations for cancer (females–breast exam; males–testicle exam).			
Public Health			
39. I walk, bike, use public transportation, or carpool whenever possible throughout the week.			
40. I recycle items such as cans, paper, glass, unused clothing, and books.			
41. I avoid polluting the air with unnecessary smoke during ozone action days.			
Safety			
42. I always use safety belts when driving or riding in a car.			
43. I always wear a helmet when roller blading or skateboarding, or riding a bike or motorcycle.			
44. Around water, I follow water safety procedures and can save myself or others from drowning.			
45. I am careful in the operation of power tools, firearms, or other dangerous equipment and follow manufacturers' recommendations regarding the use and safety of the equipment.			
46. I have installed safety features such as smoke detectors and nonskid rugs in my home.			
47. I know how to perform basic first aid measures to help others in an emergency.			
Total			

SCORING

1. Questions 1–10: Give yourself 1 point for each question you answered *yes*, 5 points for each question you answered *no*.
2. Questions 11–47: Give yourself 5 points for each question you answered *usually* (or *always*), 3 points for each *sometimes*, and 1 point for each *rarely*.
3. Add up all your points. The total is your inventory score.
4. Your score relates to the Wellness Continuum as follows.

175 and higher: You are at low risk. You are practicing many good health behaviors.

80 to 174: You are in a neutral zone. You may not be ill, but you are at risk for long-term health problems; not getting everything you could out of life.

79 or lower: You are at high risk. In what sections did you answer rarely or sometimes? Pinpoint areas that need your attention, and find ways to lower your risk.

No matter what your score, you can make changes to increase your health. Always look for ways in which you can modify behaviors to lower health risks and improve your level of wellness.

*Adapted from: *Personal Health Inventory* by Getchell, Pippin, and Varnes, "Perspectives On Health" *www.uh.edu/fitness/PPTs/personal-health-inventory.pdf*

B Appendix

EVALUATION OF STUDENT PERFORMANCE
Conducting a Physical Examination and Sample History

STUDENT: ____________________ **INSTRUCTOR:** ____________________

FIRST ATTEMPT: DATE: ________________ **SATISFACTORY** **UNSATISFACTORY**

SECOND ATTEMPT: DATE: ________________ **SATISFACTORY** **UNSATISFACTORY**

BEHAVIORS	YES	NO	COMMENTS
I. CHECK: Performs a Scene Size-Up			
*1. Determines scene safety before approaching patient.			
II. CHECK PATIENT: Performs a Primary (Initial) Assessment			
*1. Introduces self by name and level of training.			
*2. Gains patient's consent to treat.			
*3. Puts on gloves.			
*4. Checks for conditions that are an immediate threat to life (LOC, airway, breathing, circulation).			
*5. Checks skin characteristics.			
*6. **Call EMS** if life-threatening conditions exist.			
III. CARE: Secondary Assessment - Performing a Physical Examination			
*1. Performs a physical examination in an organized manner moving from head to toe.			
2. Conducts the physical examination looking and feeling for DOTS.			
*a. Checks the head.			
*b. Checks neck.			
*c. Checks shoulders and collarbones. Asks patient to shrug shoulders.			
*d. Checks the chest. Asks patient to take a deep breath.			
*e. Checks abdomen, palpating the four quadrants.			
*f. Checks the pelvis, pushing down and in on both sides.			
*g. Checks the arms and hands. Asks patient to move fingers, arms, and hands.			

BEHAVIORS	YES	NO	COMMENTS
*h. Checks the legs and feet. Asks patient to move toes, feet, ankles, and legs.			
*i. Reaches under the patient to check the back for bleeding.			
IV. CARE: Obtaining a Sample History			
*1. Asks the patient about symptoms; emergency medical responder notes any signs.			
*2. Asks patient about allergies to food, medications, environmental factors.			
*3. Asks patient if currently taking prescription or non-prescription medications.			
*4. Asks patient about pertinent past medical conditions.			
*5. Asks patient about last oral intake of food, liquids, or medications.			
*6. Asks patient what he/she was doing at the time of the illness or injury.			
V. CARE: Performing an Ongoing Assessment			
*1. States that the primary (initial) assessment will be repeated every 15 minutes for a stable patient and every 5 minutes for an unstable patient.			

EVALUATION OF STUDENT PERFORMANCE
Artificial Ventilations–Adult

STUDENT: ______________________ **INSTRUCTOR:** ______________________

FIRST ATTEMPT: DATE: ________________ **SATISFACTORY** **UNSATISFACTORY**

SECOND ATTEMPT: DATE: ________________ **SATISFACTORY** **UNSATISFACTORY**

BEHAVIORS	YES	NO	COMMENTS
I. CHECK: Performs a Scene Size-Up			
*1. Determines scene safety before approaching patient.			
II. CHECK PATIENT: Performs a Primary (Initial) Assessment			
*1. Puts on gloves.			
*2. Assesses level of consciousness.			
*3. **CALL EMS:** Patient is unconscious.			
*4. Checks for signs of life. a. Opens the airway using the head-tilt/chin-lift method. States that the jaw thrust method would be used for a patient with a suspected head, neck, or spinal injury b. Look, listens, and feels for movement and breathing for no more than 10 seconds			
*5. If not breathing, positions resuscitation mask over the patient's nose and mouth and gives two ventilations.			
*6. If the ventilations do not go in, re-tilts the head and gives two additional ventilations.			
*7. If ventilations go in, checks for carotid pulse.			
*8. Looks for any bleeding.			
III. CARE: Performs Artificial Ventilations			
*1. If the patient has a pulse but is not breathing: Begins artificial ventilations (1 ventilation every 5 seconds).			
*2. After 2 minutes of giving artificial ventilations, removes resuscitation mask. Looks for movement and rechecks pulse and breathing for no more than 10 seconds.			
*3. If there is a pulse but no movement or breathing, replaces resuscitation mask and continues giving artificial ventilation.			
*4. If there is a pulse and breathing but the victim remains unconscious, leaves the patient in a supine position until EMS arrives. Places patient in a modified H.A.IN.E.S recovery position only if the rescuer is alone and must leave the patient or if an open airway cannot be maintained due to fluid or vomit.			
****BECAUSE THIS IS A LIFE-THREATENING CONDITION, THE STUDENT MUST RECEIVE A "YES" RATING ON ALL OF THE STARRED BEHAVIORS TO PASS.**			

EVALUATION OF STUDENT PERFORMANCE
Artificial Ventilations–Child

STUDENT: ______________________ **INSTRUCTOR:** ______________________

FIRST ATTEMPT: DATE: ________________ **SATISFACTORY** **UNSATISFACTORY**

SECOND ATTEMPT: DATE: ________________ **SATISFACTORY** **UNSATISFACTORY**

BEHAVIORS	YES	NO	COMMENTS
I. CHECK: Performs a Scene Size-Up			
*1. Determines scene safety before approaching patient.			
II. CHECK PATIENT: Performs a Primary (Initial) Assessment			
*1. Puts on gloves.			
*2. Assesses level of consciousness.			
*3. **CALL EMS:** Patient is unconscious.			
*4. Checks for signs of life. a. Opens the airway using the head-tilt/chin-lift method. States that the jaw thrust method would be used for a patient with a suspected head, neck, or spinal injury. b. Look, listens, and feels for movement and breathing for no more than 10 seconds.			
*5. If not breathing, positions the resuscitation mask over the patient's nose and mouth and gives two ventilations.			
*6. If ventilations do not go in, re-tilts the head and tries to give two additional ventilations.			
*7. If ventilations go in, checks for carotid pulse for no more than 10 seconds.			
*8. Looks for any bleeding.			
III. CARE: Performs Rescue Breathing			
*1. If the child has a pulse but is not breathing: Begins artificial ventilations (1 ventilation every 3 seconds).			
*2. After 2 minutes of giving artificial ventilations, removes resuscitation mask. Looks for movement and rechecks pulse and breathing for no more than 10 seconds.			
*3. If there is a pulse but no movement or breathing, replaces resuscitation mask and continues giving artificial ventilations			
*4. If there is a pulse and breathing but the patient remains unconscious, leaves the patient in a supine position until EMS arrives. Places patient in a modified H.A.IN.E.S recovery position only if the rescuer is alone and must leave the patient or if an open airway cannot be maintained due to fluid or vomit.			
****BECAUSE THIS IS A LIFE-THREATENING CONDITION, THE STUDENT MUST RECEIVE A "YES" RATING ON ALL OF THE STARRED BEHAVIORS TO PASS.**			

EVALUATION OF STUDENT PERFORMANCE
Artificial Ventilations–Infant

STUDENT: ______________________ **INSTRUCTOR:** ______________________

FIRST ATTEMPT: DATE: ________________ **SATISFACTORY** **UNSATISFACTORY**

SECOND ATTEMPT: DATE: ________________ **SATISFACTORY** **UNSATISFACTORY**

BEHAVIORS	YES	NO	COMMENTS
I. CHECK: Performs a Scene Size-Up			
*1. Determines scene safety before approaching patient.			
II. CHECK PATIENT: Performs a Primary (Initial) Assessment			
*1. Puts on gloves.			
*2. Assesses level of consciousness.			
*3. **CALL EMS:** Patient is unconscious.			
*4. Checks for signs of life. a. Opens the airway using the head-tilt/chin-lift method. States that the jaw thrust method would be used for a patient with a suspected head, neck, or spinal injury. b. Look, listens, and feels for movement and breathing for no more than 10 seconds.			
*5. If not breathing, positions the resuscitation mask over the patient's nose and mouth and gives two ventilations.			
*6. If breaths do not go in, re-tilts the head and tries to give two additional ventilations.			
*7. If breaths go in, checks for brachial pulse.			
*8. Looks for severe bleeding.			
III. CARE: Performs Rescue Breathing			
*1. If a pulse is present but is not breathing: Begins artificial ventilations (1 breath every 3 seconds) using a resuscitation mask.			
*2. After 2 minutes of giving artificial ventilations removes resuscitation mask. Looks for movement and rechecks pulse and breathing for no more than 10 seconds.			
*3. If there is a pulse but no movement or breathing, replaces resuscitation mask and continues giving artificial ventilations.			
*4. If there is a pulse and breathing but the infant remains unconscious, leaves the infant in a supine position until EMS arrives. The infant can also be placed in a recovery position by laying the infant face-down along the forearm of the emergency medical responder. The emergency medical responder's other hand is used to support the infant's head and neck.			
****BECAUSE THIS IS A LIFE-THREATENING CONDITION, THE STUDENT MUST RECEIVE A "YES" RATING ON ALL OF THE STARRED BEHAVIORS TO PASS.**			

EVALUATION OF STUDENT PERFORMANCE
Foreign Body Airway Obstruction (FBAO)—Unconscious Adult

STUDENT: ______________________ **INSTRUCTOR:** ______________________

FIRST ATTEMPT: DATE: ______________________ **SATISFACTORY** **UNSATISFACTORY**

SECOND ATTEMPT: DATE: ______________________ **SATISFACTORY** **UNSATISFACTORY**

BEHAVIORS	YES	NO	COMMENTS
I. CHECK: Performs a Scene Size-Up			
*1. Determines scene safety before approaching patient.			
II. CHECK PATIENT: Performs a Primary (Initial) Assessment			
*1. Puts on gloves.			
*2. Assesses level of consciousness.			
*3. **CALL EMS:** Patient is unconscious.			
*4. Checks for signs of life. a. Opens the airway using head- tilt/chin-lift method. States that the jaw thrust method would be used for a patient with a suspected head, neck, or spinal injury. b. Looks, listens, and feels for movement and breathing for no more than 10 seconds.			
*5. If the victim is not breathing, places resuscitation mask over the patient's nose and mouth and gives two ventilations.			
*6. If ventilations do not go in, re-tilts the head and tries to give two additional ventilations.			
*7. If ventilations go in, checks for a carotid pulse for no more than 10 seconds.			
*8. Looks for severe bleeding.			
*9. If ventilations do not go in, assumes there is an airway obstruction.			
III. CARE: Relieving an Airway Obstruction			
*1. Removes resuscitation mask.			
*2. Places two hands on the center of the patient's chest and gives 30 chest compressions at a depth of at least 2 inches			
*3. Looks inside the patient's mouth. Performs finger sweep only if object is seen, using index finger and hooking motion.			
*4. Opens the airway, replaces the resuscitation mask, and attempts to give two ventilations.			

BEHAVIORS	YES	NO	COMMENTS
III. CARE: Relieving an Airway Obstruction			
*5. If ventilations do not go in, repeats steps 2–4.			
*6. If ventilations go in, checks for breathing and a pulse.			
*7. If there is a pulse but not breathing, begins giving artificial ventilations, 1 ventilation every 5 seconds			
*8. If there is a pulse and breathing, but the patient remains unconscious, leaves the patient in a supine position until EMS arrives. Places patient in a modified H.A.IN.E.S recovery position only if the rescuer is alone and must leave the patient or if an open airway cannot be maintained due to fluid or vomit.			
****BECAUSE THIS IS A LIFE-THREATENING CONDITION, THE STUDENT MUST RECEIVE A "YES" RATING ON ALL OF THE STARRED BEHAVIORS TO PASS.**			

EVALUATION OF STUDENT PERFORMANCE
Foreign Body Airway Obstruction (FBAO)—Unconscious Child

STUDENT: ______________________ **INSTRUCTOR:** ______________________

FIRST ATTEMPT: DATE: ________________ **SATISFACTORY** **UNSATISFACTORY**

SECOND ATTEMPT: DATE: ________________ **SATISFACTORY** **UNSATISFACTORY**

BEHAVIORS	YES	NO	COMMENTS
I. CHECK: Performs a Scene Size-Up			
1. Determines scene safety before approaching patient.			
II. CHECK PATIENT: Performs a Primary (Initial) Assessment			
*1. Puts on gloves.			
*2. Assesses level of consciousness.			
*3. **CALL EMS:** Patient is unconscious.			
*4. Checks for signs of life. a. Opens the airway using the head-tilt/chin-lift method. States that the jaw thrust method would be used for a patient with a suspected head, neck, or spinal injury. b. Looks, listens, and feels for movement and breathing for no more than 10 seconds.			
*5. If the patient is not breathing, places the resuscitation mask over the patient's nose and mouth and gives two ventilations.			
*6. If ventilations do not go in, re-tilts the head and tries to give two additional ventilations.			
*7. If ventilations go in, checks for a carotid pulse.			
*8. Looks for severe bleeding.			
*9. If ventilations do not go in, assumes there is an airway obstruction.			
III. CARE: Relieving an Airway Obstruction			
*1. Removes the resuscitation mask.			
*2. Places two hands on the center of the chest and gives 30 chest compressions at a depth of about 2 inches.			
*3. Looks inside the child's mouth. Performs a finger sweep if an object is seen using the little finger and hooking motion.			
*4. Opens the airway and attempts to give two ventilations.			

BEHAVIORS	YES	NO	COMMENTS
III. CARE: Relieving an Airway Obstruction			
*5. If ventilations do not go in, repeat steps 2–4.			
*6. If ventilations go in, checks for breathing and a pulse.			
*7. If there is a pulse but not breathing, begins giving artificial ventilations, 1 ventilation every 3 seconds.			
*8. If there is a pulse and breathing but the patient remains unconscious, leaves the patient in a supine position until EMS arrives. Places patient in a modified H.A.IN.E.S. recovery position only if the rescuer is alone and must leave the patient or if an open airway cannot be maintained due to fluid or vomit.			
****BECAUSE THIS IS A LIFE-THREATENING CONDITION, THE STUDENT MUST RECEIVE A "YES" RATING ON ALL OF THE STARRED BEHAVIORS TO PASS.**			

EVALUATION OF STUDENT PERFORMANCE
Foreign Body Airway Obstruction (FBAO)—Unconscious Infant

STUDENT: ______________________________ **INSTRUCTOR:** ______________________

FIRST ATTEMPT: DATE: ____________________ **SATISFACTORY** **UNSATISFACTORY**

SECOND ATTEMPT: DATE: ____________________ **SATISFACTORY** **UNSATISFACTORY**

BEHAVIORS	YES	NO	COMMENTS
I. CHECK: Performs a Scene Size-Up			
*1. Determines scene safety before approaching patient.			
II. CHECK PATIENT: Performs an Initial Assessment			
*1. Puts on gloves.			
*2. Assesses level of consciousness.			
*3. **CALL EMS:** Patient is unconscious.			
*4. Checks for signs of life. a. Opens the airway using the head-tilt/chin-lift method. b. Look, listens, and feels for movement and breathing for no more than 10 seconds.			
*5. Places the resuscitation mask over the patient's nose and mouth and gives two ventilations.			
*6. If ventilations do not go in, re-tilts the head and tries to give two additional ventilations.			
*7. If ventilations go in, checks for a brachial pulse for no more than 10 seconds.			
*8. Looks for severe bleeding.			
*9. If ventilations do not go in, assumes there is an airway obstruction.			
III. CARE: Relieving an Airway Obstruction			
*1. Removes the resuscitation mask.			
*2. Places one hand on the infant's forehead to maintain an open airway.			
*3. Places pad of index finger on the imaginary line between the nipples.			
*4. Places pads of two fingers next to the index finger on the sternum.			

BEHAVIORS	YES	NO	COMMENTS
III. CARE: Relieving a Foreign Body Airway Obstruction			
*5. Lifts index finger off the chest.			
*6. Gives 30 chest compressions using the pads of the middle and ring fingers. Depresses the chest about 1 ½ inches.			
*7. Opens the mouth and looks for object. If seen, performs a finger sweep with the little finger using a hooking motion.			
*8. Opens the airway, replaces the resuscitation mask, and attempts to give two ventilations.			
*9. If ventilations do not go in, repeat steps 2–7.			
*10. If ventilations go in, checks for breathing and a pulse.			
*11. If there is a pulse but not breathing, begins giving artificial ventilations, 1 ventilation every 3 seconds.			
*12. If there is a pulse and breathing but the infant remains unconscious, leaves the infant in a supine position until EMS arrives. The infant can also be placed in a recovery position by laying the infant face-down along the forearm of the emergency medical responder. The emergency medical responder's other hand is used to support the infant's head and neck.			
****BECAUSE THIS IS A LIFE-THREATENING CONDITION, THE STUDENT MUST RECEIVE A "YES" RATING ON ALL OF THE STARRED BEHAVIORS TO PASS.**			

EVALUATION OF STUDENT PERFORMANCE
CPR–Adult

STUDENT: ______________________ **INSTRUCTOR:** ______________________

FIRST ATTEMPT: DATE: ______________ **SATISFACTORY** **UNSATISFACTORY**

SECOND ATTEMPT: DATE: ______________ **SATISFACTORY** **UNSATISFACTORY**

BEHAVIORS	YES	NO	COMMENTS
I. CHECK: Performs a Scene Size-Up			
1. Determines scene safety before approaching patient.			
II. CHECK PATIENT: Performs a Primary (Initial) Assessment			
*1. Puts on gloves.			
*2. Assesses level of consciousness.			
*3. **CALL EMS:** Patient is unconscious.			
*4. Checks for signs of life. a. Opens airway using head- tilt/chin-lift method. States that the jaw thrust would be used for a patient suspected of having a head, neck, or spinal injury. b. Looks, listens, and feels for movement and breathing for no more than 10 seconds.			
*5. If not breathing, places resuscitation mask over patient's nose and mouth and gives two ventilations.			
*6. If the ventilations do not go in, re-tilts head and tries to give two additional ventilations.			
*7. If ventilations go in, checks for a carotid pulse. **States that in a witnessed sudden collapse of an adult, quickly check for the presence of breathing and a pulse. If neither is present, begin chest compressions. The two initial ventilations are eliminated.**			
*8. Looks for any bleeding.			
*9. If there is no pulse and no breathing, states that CPR is needed.			
III. CARE: Performs CPR			
*1. Places the patient on a firm, flat surface.			
*2. Positions self on knees beside the patient's chest.			
*3. Finds correct hand placement: a. Places the heel of the dominant hand on the center of the patient's chest. b. Places the other hand directly on top, interlocking fingers. c. With hands in place, positions self so that shoulders are directly over hands, arms straight, and elbows locked.			

BEHAVIORS	YES	NO	COMMENTS
III. CARE: Performs CPR			
*4. Begins compressions using the heels of both hands, compressing the sternum at least 2 inches.			
*5. Counting out loud, compresses the chest 30 times, at a rate of 100 compressions per minute.			
*6. Following chest compressions, gives two ventilations.			
*7. Repeat cycles of 30 compressions and two ventilations until: • Another trained responder takes over • An AED is ready to use • You're too exhausted to continue • The scene becomes unsafe • You notice an obvious sign of life • You are presented with a valid DNR order • More advanced medical personnel take over.			
*8. If there is a pulse and breathing but the patient remains unconscious, leave the patient in a supine position until EMS arrives. Places patient in a modified H.A.IN.E.S. recovery position only if the rescuer is alone and must leave the patient or if an open airway cannot be maintained due to fluid or vomit.			
****BECAUSE THIS IS A LIFE-THREATENING CONDITION, THE STUDENT MUST RECEIVE A "YES" RATING ON ALL OF THE STARRED BEHAVIORS TO PASS.**			

EVALUATION OF STUDENT PERFORMANCE
CPR–Child

STUDENT: ______________________ **INSTRUCTOR:** ______________________

FIRST ATTEMPT: DATE: ________________ **SATISFACTORY** **UNSATISFACTORY**

SECOND ATTEMPT: DATE: ________________ **SATISFACTORY** **UNSATISFACTORY**

BEHAVIORS	YES	NO	COMMENTS
I. CHECK: Performs a Scene Size-Up			
*1. Determines scene safety before approaching patient.			
II. CHECK PATIENT: Performs a Primary (Initial) Assessment			
*1. Puts on gloves.			
*2. Assesses level of consciousness.			
*3. **CALL EMS:** Patient is unconscious.			
*4. Checks for signs of life. a. Opens airway using head-tilt/chin-lift method. States that the jaw thrust method would be used for a patient with a suspected head, neck, or spinal injury b. Looks, listens, and feels for movement and breathing for no more than 10 seconds..			
*5. If not breathing, places resuscitation mask over patient's nose and mouth and gives two ventilations.			
*6. If ventilations do not go in, re-tilts the head and tries to give two additional ventilations.			
*7. If ventilations go in, checks for a carotid pulse.			
*8. Looks for any bleeding.			
*9. If there is no pulse and no breathing, states that CPR is needed.			
III. CARE: Performs CPR			
*1. Positions child face up on a firm, flat surface.			
*2. Positions self on knees next to the child's chest.			
*3. Finds correct hand placement: a. Places the heel of the dominant hand on the center of the child's chest. b. Places the other hand directly on top, interlocking fingers.			
*4. With hands in place, positions self so that shoulders are directly over hands, arms are straight, and elbows locked.			
*5. Begins compressions using the heels of both hands, compressing the chest about 2 inches.			

BEHAVIORS	YES	NO	COMMENTS
III. CARE: Performs CPR			
*6. Counting out loud, compresses the chest 30 times, at a rate of 100 compressions per minute.			
*7. Following chest compressions, gives two ventilations.			
*8. Repeat cycles of 30 compressions and two ventilations until: • Another trained responder takes over • An AED is ready to use • You're too exhausted to continue • The scene becomes unsafe • You notice an obvious sign of life • You are presented with a valid DNR order • More advanced medical personnel take over.			
*9. If there is a pulse and breathing but the patient remains unconscious, leave the patient in a supine position until EMS arrives. Places patient in a modified H.A.IN.E.S. recovery position only if the rescuer is alone and must leave the patient or if an open airway cannot be maintained due to fluid or vomit.			
****BECAUSE THIS IS A LIFE-THREATENING CONDITION, THE STUDENT MUST RECEIVE A "YES" RATING ON ALL OF THE STARRED BEHAVIORS TO PASS.**			

EVALUATION OF STUDENT PERFORMANCE
CPR–Infant

STUDENT: ______________________ **INSTRUCTOR:** ______________________

FIRST ATTEMPT: DATE: ______________ **SATISFACTORY** **UNSATISFACTORY**

SECOND ATTEMPT: DATE: ______________ **SATISFACTORY** **UNSATISFACTORY**

BEHAVIORS	YES	NO	COMMENTS
I. CHECK: Performs a Scene Size-Up			
*1. Determines scene safety before approaching patient.			
II. CHECK PATIENT: Performs A Primary (Initial) Assessment			
*1. Puts on gloves.			
*2. Assesses level of consciousness.			
*3. **CALL EMS:** Patient is unconscious.			
*4. Checks for signs of life. a. Opens the airway using head-tilt/chin-lift method. States that the jaw thrust method would be used for a patient with a suspected head, neck, or back injury. b. Looks, listens, and feels for movement and breathing for no more than 10 seconds.			
*5. If there is no breathing, places resuscitation mask over patient's nose and mouth and gives two ventilations.			
*6. If ventilations do not go in, re-tilts the head and tries to give two additional ventilations.			
*7. If ventilations go in, checks for a brachial pulse.			
*8. Looks for any bleeding.			
*9. If there is no pulse, states that CPR is needed.			
III. CARE: Performs CPR			
*1. Positions the infant face up on a firm, flat surface.			
*2. Stands or kneels facing the infant from the side.			
*3. Keeps one hand on the infant's head to maintain an open airway and uses the fingers of the other hand to give compressions.			
*4. Finds correct finger placement. a. Places pad of index finger on the imaginary line between the nipples. b. Places the pads of two fingers next to the index finger on the sternum. c. Lifts index finger off the chest.			
*5. Begins compressions using the pads of the middle and ring fingers and compresses the chest about 1½ inches.			

BEHAVIORS	YES	NO	COMMENTS
III. CARE: Performs CPR			
*6. Counting out loud, compresses the chest 30 times, at a rate of 100 compressions per minute.			
*7. Following chest compressions, gives two ventilations.			
*8. Repeat cycles of 30 compressions and two ventilations until: • Another trained responder takes over • You're too exhausted to continue • Scene becomes unsafe • You notice an obvious sign of life • An AED is ready to use • You are presented with a valid DNR order • More advanced medical personnel take over.			
*9. If there is a pulse and breathing but the infant remains unconscious, leave the infant in a supine position until EMS arrives. The infant can be placed in a recovery position by laying the infant face-down along the forearm of the emergency medical responder. The emergency medical responder's other hand is used to support the infant's head and neck.			
****BECAUSE THIS IS A LIFE-THREATENING CONDITION, THE STUDENT MUST RECEIVE A "YES" RATING ON ALL OF THE STARRED BEHAVIORS TO PASS.**			

EVALUATION OF STUDENT PERFORMANCE
Two-Rescuer CPR–Adult

STUDENT: ______________________ **INSTRUCTOR:** ______________________

FIRST ATTEMPT: DATE: ________________ **SATISFACTORY** **UNSATISFACTORY**

SECOND ATTEMPT: DATE: ________________ **SATISFACTORY** **UNSATISFACTORY**

BEHAVIORS	YES	NO	COMMENTS
I. CHECK: Scene Size-Up and Primary (Initial) Assessment Performed By Rescuer 1.			
*1. **Rescuer 2** identifies self by name and level of training.			
*2. **CALL EMS: Rescuer 2** asks if EMS has been activated. If EMS has not been activated, Rescuer 2 does so.			
II. CARE: 2-Rescuer CPR			
*1. **Rescuer 1** completes a cycle of 30 compressions and two ventilations.			
*2. When **Rescuer 1** moves to the head to give the two ventilations, **Rescuer 2** gets hands in position to start compressions.			
*3. **Rescuer 2** gives 30 compressions and **Rescuer 1** follows by giving two ventilations.			
*4. After 2 minutes of continuous CPR, **Rescuer 2** calls for a position change.			
III. CARE: Changing Positions			
*1. **Rescuer 2** (The person doing the compressions) calls for a position change by substituting the word "change" for the last compression.			
*2. a. **Compressor to ventilator:** the person doing the compressions completes the compression cycle and moves quickly to the patient's head to give ventilations. b. **Ventilator to compressor:** the person giving the ventilations completes the two ventilations, moves quickly to the patient's chest and begins compressions.			
*3. Changes position after every 2 minutes of CPR.			

EVALUATION OF STUDENT PERFORMANCE
Two-Rescuer CPR–Child and Infant

STUDENT: ______________________ **INSTRUCTOR:** ______________________

FIRST ATTEMPT: DATE: ________________ **SATISFACTORY** **UNSATISFACTORY**

SECOND ATTEMPT: DATE: ________________ **SATISFACTORY** **UNSATISFACTORY**

BEHAVIORS	YES	NO	COMMENTS
I. CHECK: Scene Size-Up and Primary (Initial) Assessment Performed By Rescuer 1.			
*1. **Rescuer 2** identifies self by name and level of training.			
*2. **CALL EMS: Rescuer 2** asks if EMS has been activated. If EMS has not been activated, Rescuer 2 does so.			
II. CARE: 2-Rescuer CPR			
*1. **Rescuer 1** completes a cycle of 15 compressions and two ventilations.			
*2. When **Rescuer 1** moves to the head to give the two ventilations, **Rescuer 2** gets hands in position to start compressions.			
*3. **Rescuer 2** gives 15 compressions and **Rescuer 1** follows by giving two ventilations.			
*4. After 2 minutes of continuous CPR, **Rescuer 2** calls for a position change.			
III. CARE: Changing Positions			
*1. **Rescuer 2** (The person doing the compressions) calls for a position change by substituting the word "change" for the last compression.			
*2. a. **Compressor to ventilator:** the person doing the compressions completes the compression cycle and moves quickly to the patient's head to give ventilations. b. **Ventilator to compressor:** the person giving the ventilations completes the two ventilations, moves quickly to the patient's chest and begins compressions.			
*3. Changes position after every 2 minutes of CPR.			

EVALUATION OF STUDENT PERFORMANCE
Using an AED with CPR in Progress–Adult, Child, Infant

STUDENT: ______________________ **INSTRUCTOR:** ______________________

FIRST ATTEMPT: DATE: ______________________ **SATISFACTORY** **UNSATISFACTORY**

SECOND ATTEMPT: DATE: ______________________ **SATISFACTORY** **UNSATISFACTORY**

BEHAVIORS	YES	NO	COMMENTS
I. CHECK: Scene Size-Up and Primary (Initial) Assessment Performed By Rescuer 1.			
*1. **Rescuer 2** identifies self by name and level of training. States an AED is available.			
*2. **CALL EMS: Rescuer 2** verifies that EMS has been called.			
II. CARE: Using an AED			
1. **Rescuer 2** opens the AED and turns the power on. **Rescuer 1** continues CPR.			
2. **Rescuer 2** wipes the chest dry and shaves the area for pad placement if necessary.			
3. **Rescuer 2** places the AED pad on the patient's bare, dry chest. Places one pad on upper right side of the chest and the second pad on the left side of the chest beneath the breast. **For a child (ages 1–8) or an infant, states that either a pediatric AED or pediatric cables must be used. Places one pad on the center of the child's or infant's chest and the second pad on the center of the child's or infant's back, between the shoulder blades.			
4. **Rescuer 2** plugs the electrode connector into the AED.			
5. **Rescuer 2** now instructs **Rescuer 1** to stop CPR.			
6. **Rescuer 2** allows the AED to analyze the patient's heart rhythm. Gives the command, "Do not touch the patient"			
7. If shock is advised: a. **Rescuer 2** tells everyone to "stand clear" of the victim. b. **Rescuer 2** presses the shock button.			
8. After the shock is delivered or if no shock is advised: **Rescuer 2** tells **Rescuer 1** to give five cycles of CPR (about 2 minutes). The AED will re-analyze the patient's heart rhythm every 2 minutes.			

BEHAVIORS	YES	NO	COMMENTS
II. CARE: Using an AED			
9. If at any time obvious signs of life are noted, stop CPR, and leave the patient in a supine position and monitor the ABCs until EMS arrives. Place the patient in a modified H.A.IN.E.S. recovery position only if the rescuer is alone and must leave the patient or if an open airway cannot be maintained due to fluid or vomit. An infant may be placed in a recovery position by laying the infant along the forearm of the emergency medical responder. The emergency medical responder's other hand is used to support the infant's head and neck.			

EVALUATION OF STUDENT PERFORMANCE
Controlling External Bleeding

STUDENT: ______________________ **INSTRUCTOR:** ______________________

FIRST ATTEMPT: DATE: ______________ **SATISFACTORY** **UNSATISFACTORY**

SECOND ATTEMPT: DATE: ______________ **SATISFACTORY** **UNSATISFACTORY**

BEHAVIORS	YES	NO	COMMENTS
I. CHECK: Performs a Scene Size-Up			
1. Determines scene safety before approaching patient.			
II. CHECK PATIENT: Determines Extent of External Bleeding			
*1. Identifies self by name and level of training.			
*2. Gains consent from the patient.			
*3. **CALL EMS** if necessary.			
III. CARE: Controlling External Bleeding			
*1. Puts on gloves.			
*2. Covers open wound with a 4x4 gauze dressing. Applies direct pressure with palm of the hand over the dressing.			
*3. Covers the 4x4 dressing with a pressure bandage.			
*4. Secures the pressure bandage by tying or taping it.			
*5. Checks circulation of the extremity below the level of the wound.			
*6. States that if bleeding continues, another pressure bandage would be applied over the top of the first one.			

EVALUATION OF STUDENT PERFORMANCE
Splinting

STUDENT: ______________________ **INSTRUCTOR:** ______________________

FIRST ATTEMPT: DATE: ________________ **SATISFACTORY** **UNSATISFACTORY**

SECOND ATTEMPT: DATE: ________________ **SATISFACTORY** **UNSATISFACTORY**

BEHAVIORS	**YES**	**NO**	**COMMENTS**
I. CHECK: Performs a Scene Size-Up			
1. Determines scene safety before approaching patient.			
II. CHECK PATIENT: Inspects the Affected Area for DOTs			
*1. Identifies self by name and level of training.			
*2. Gains consent from the patient.			
*3. **CALL EMS** if necessary.			
III. CARE: Applies a Splint			
*1. Puts on gloves.			
*2. Covers any open wounds with a dressing before applying the splint.			
*3. Supports the injury site and minimizes movement until splinting is completed.			
*4. If the injury involves an extremity, checks circulation and sensation below the injury.			
*5. Selects the appropriate splint and immobilizes the joint above and below the injury site using cravats.			
*6. States that the limb would be splinted in the position in which it was found.			
*7. If applicable, correctly fashions a sling from a cravat.			
*8. Re-checks the circulation of the affected extremity following splinting.			
*9. States that ice would be applied after the splinting.			
*10. Elevates the extremity if possible.			

C Appendix

CLEARING A FBAO—CONSCIOUS ADULT AND CHILD

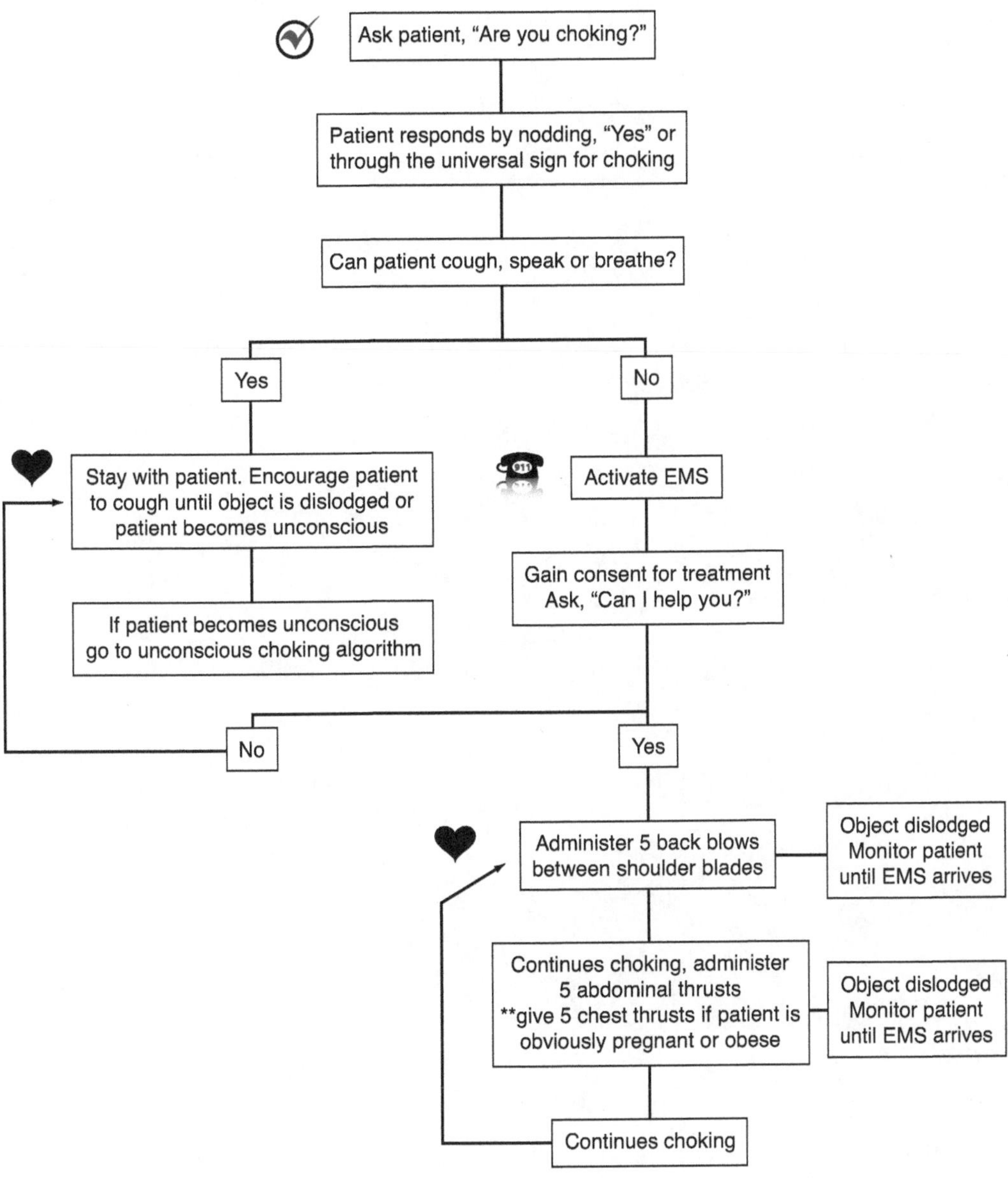
Ask patient, "Are you choking?"
Patient responds by nodding, "Yes" or through the universal sign for choking
Can patient cough, speak or breathe?
Yes
No
Stay with patient. Encourage patient to cough until object is dislodged or patient becomes unconscious
If patient becomes unconscious go to unconscious choking algorithm
Activate EMS
Gain consent for treatment Ask, "Can I help you?"
No
Yes
Administer 5 back blows between shoulder blades
Object dislodged Monitor patient until EMS arrives
Continues choking, administer 5 abdominal thrusts **give 5 chest thrusts if patient is obviously pregnant or obese
Object dislodged Monitor patient until EMS arrives
Continues choking

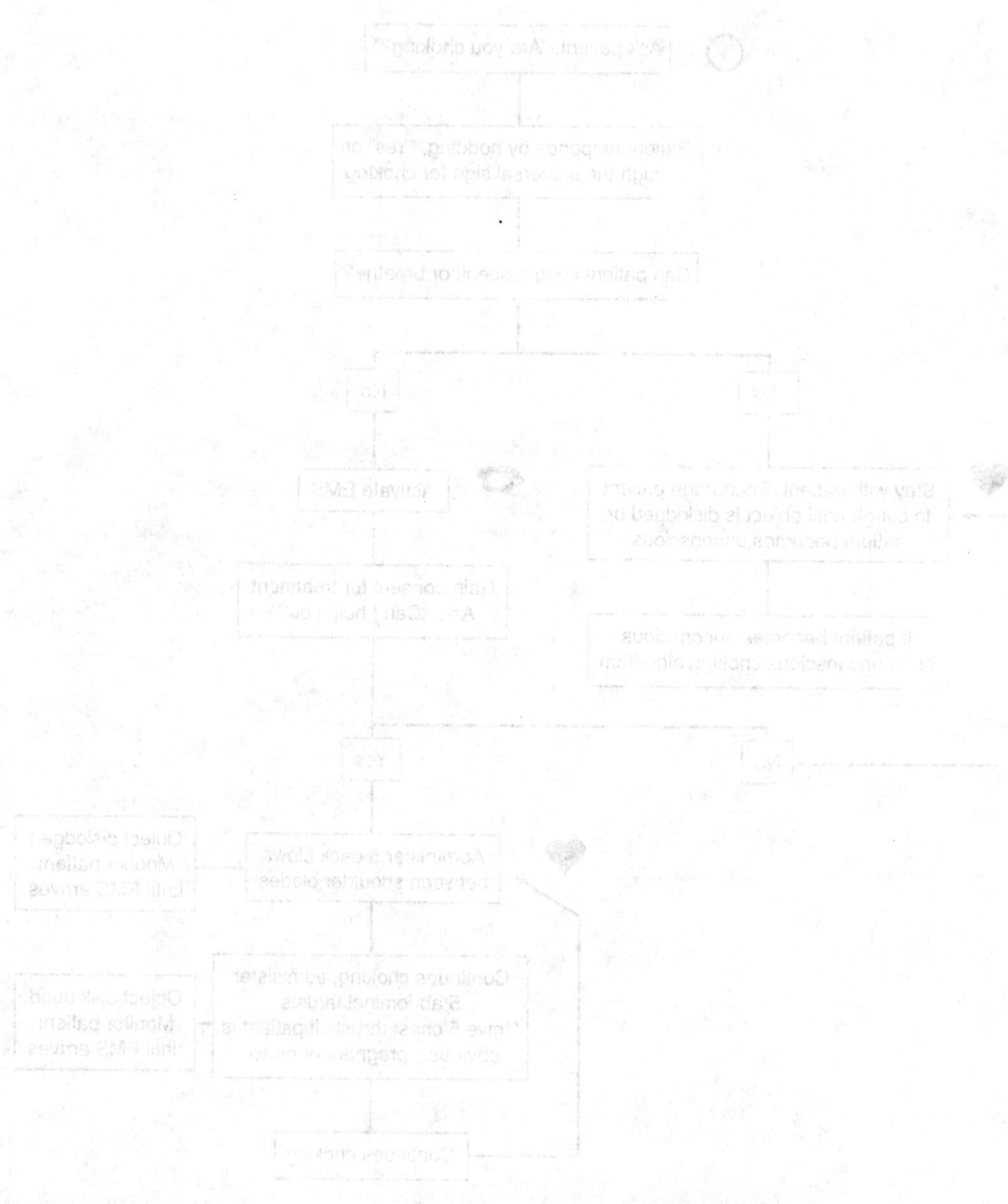

CLEARING A FBAO—CONSCIOUS INFANT

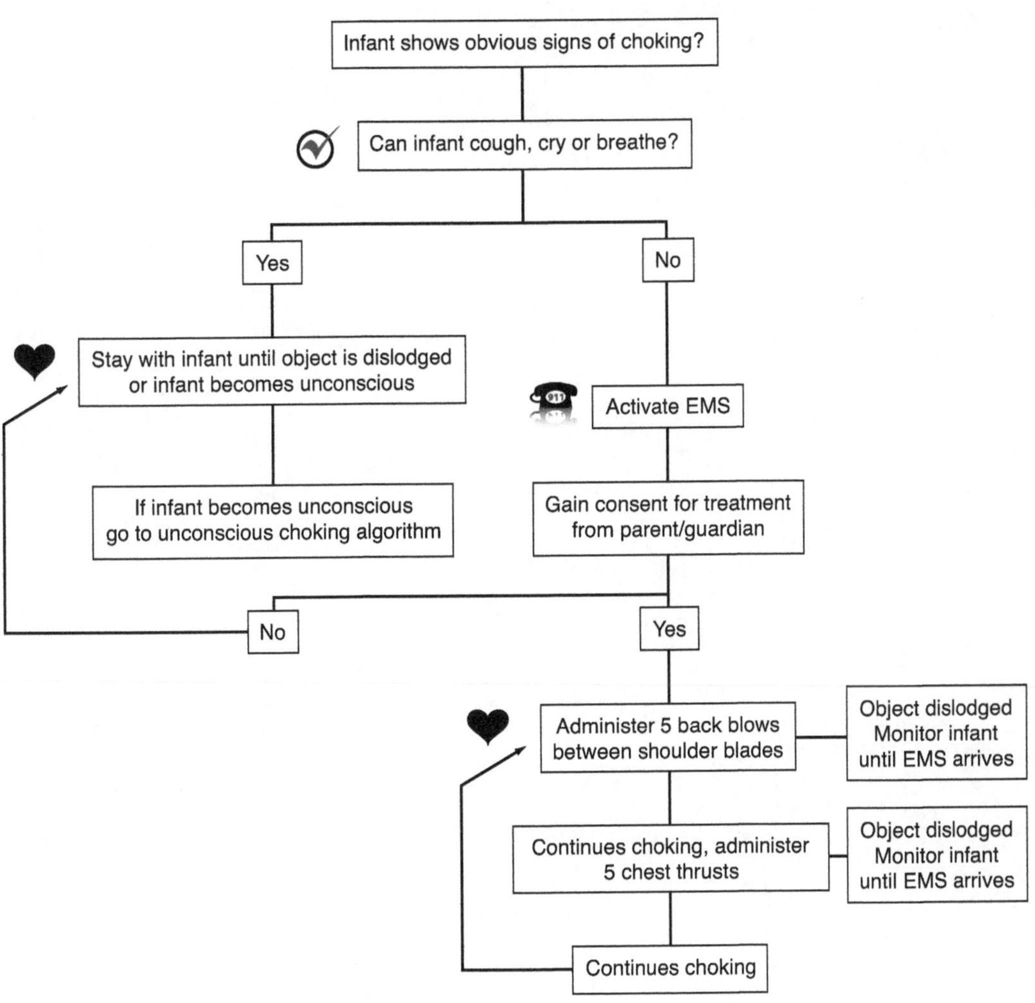

Infant shows obvious signs of choking?
Can infant cough, cry or breathe?
Yes
No
Stay with infant until object is dislodged or infant becomes unconscious
Activate EMS
If infant becomes unconscious go to unconscious choking algorithm
Gain consent for treatment from parent/guardian
No
Yes
Administer 5 back blows between shoulder blades
Object dislodged Monitor infant until EMS arrives
Continues choking, administer 5 chest thrusts
Object dislodged Monitor infant until EMS arrives
Continues choking

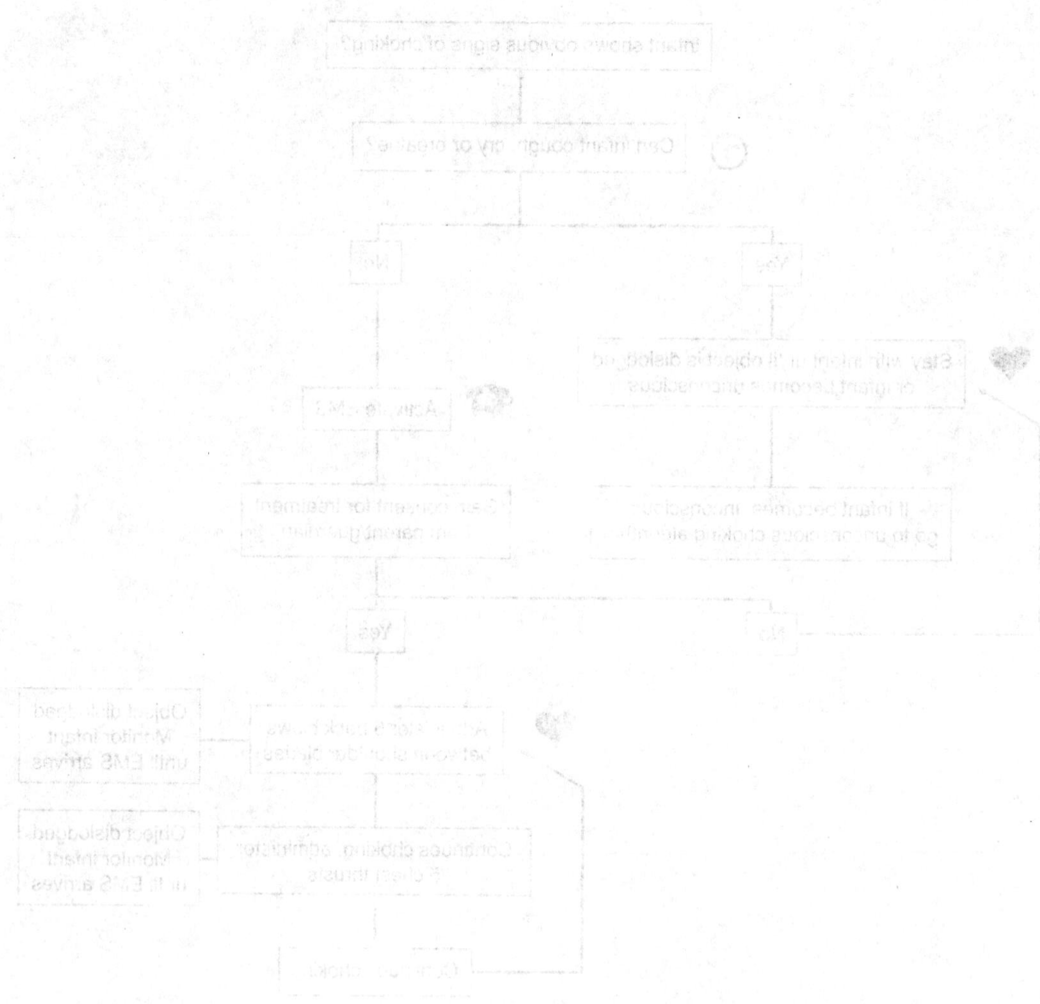

CLEARING A FBAO—UNCONSCIOUS ADULT AND CHILD

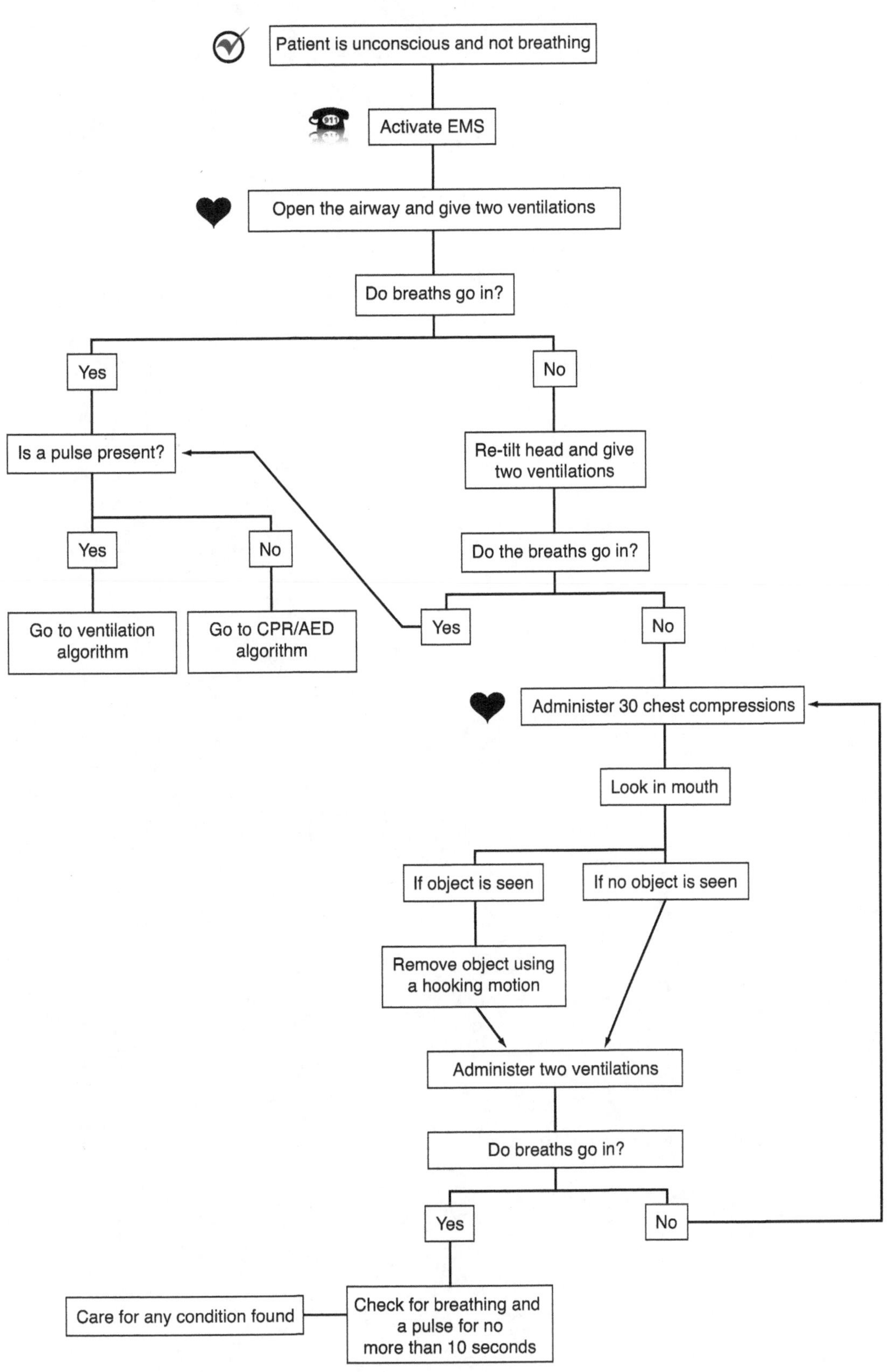
Patient is unconscious and not breathing
911
Activate EMS
Open the airway and give two ventilations
Do breaths go in?
Yes
No
Is a pulse present?
Re-tilt head and give two ventilations
Yes
No
Do the breaths go in?
Go to ventilation algorithm
Go to CPR/AED algorithm
Yes
No
Administer 30 chest compressions
Look in mouth
If object is seen
If no object is seen
Remove object using a hooking motion
Administer two ventilations
Do breaths go in?
Yes
No
Care for any condition found
Check for breathing and a pulse for no more than 10 seconds

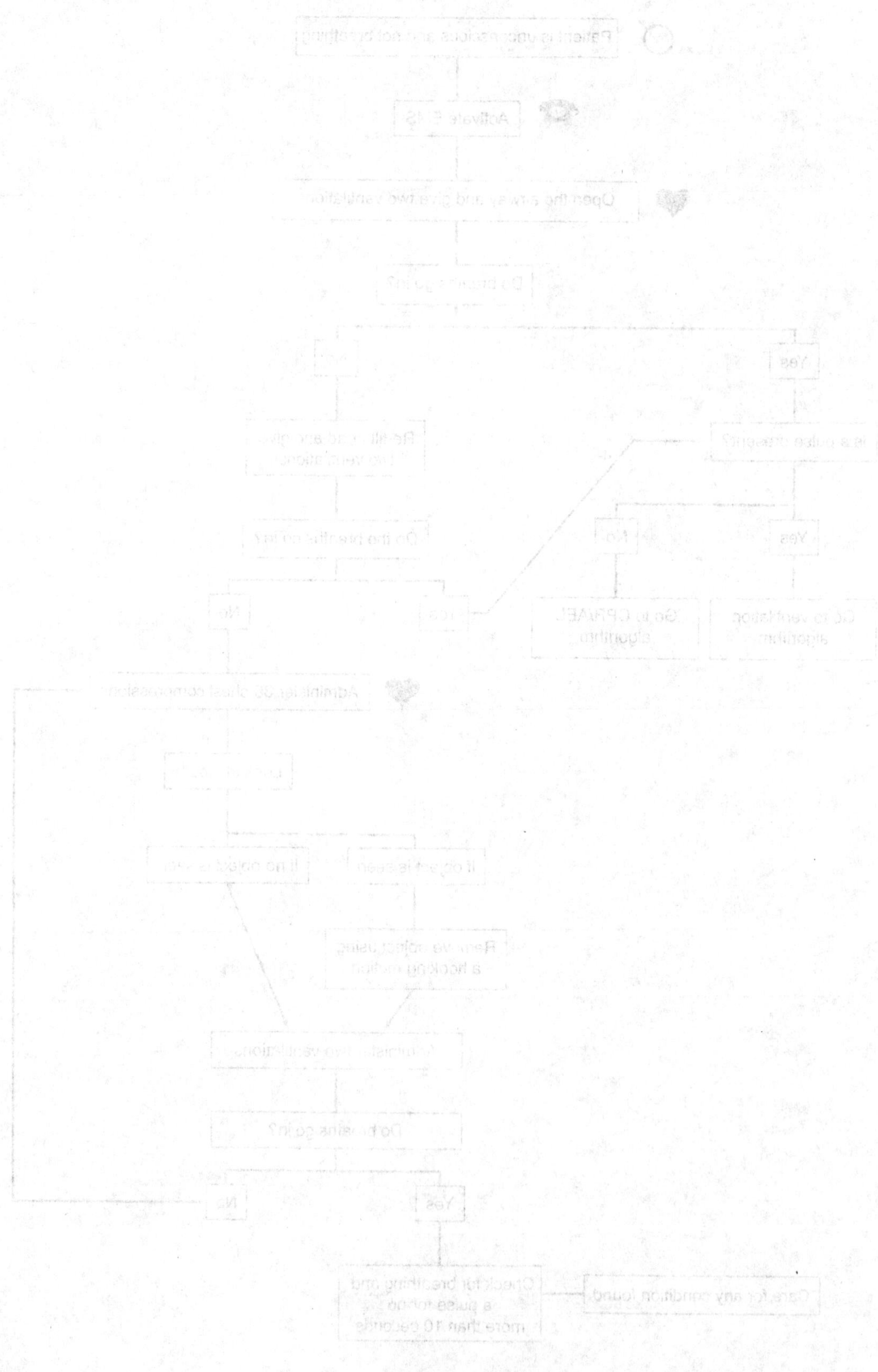

CLEARING A FBAO—UNCONSCIOUS INFANT

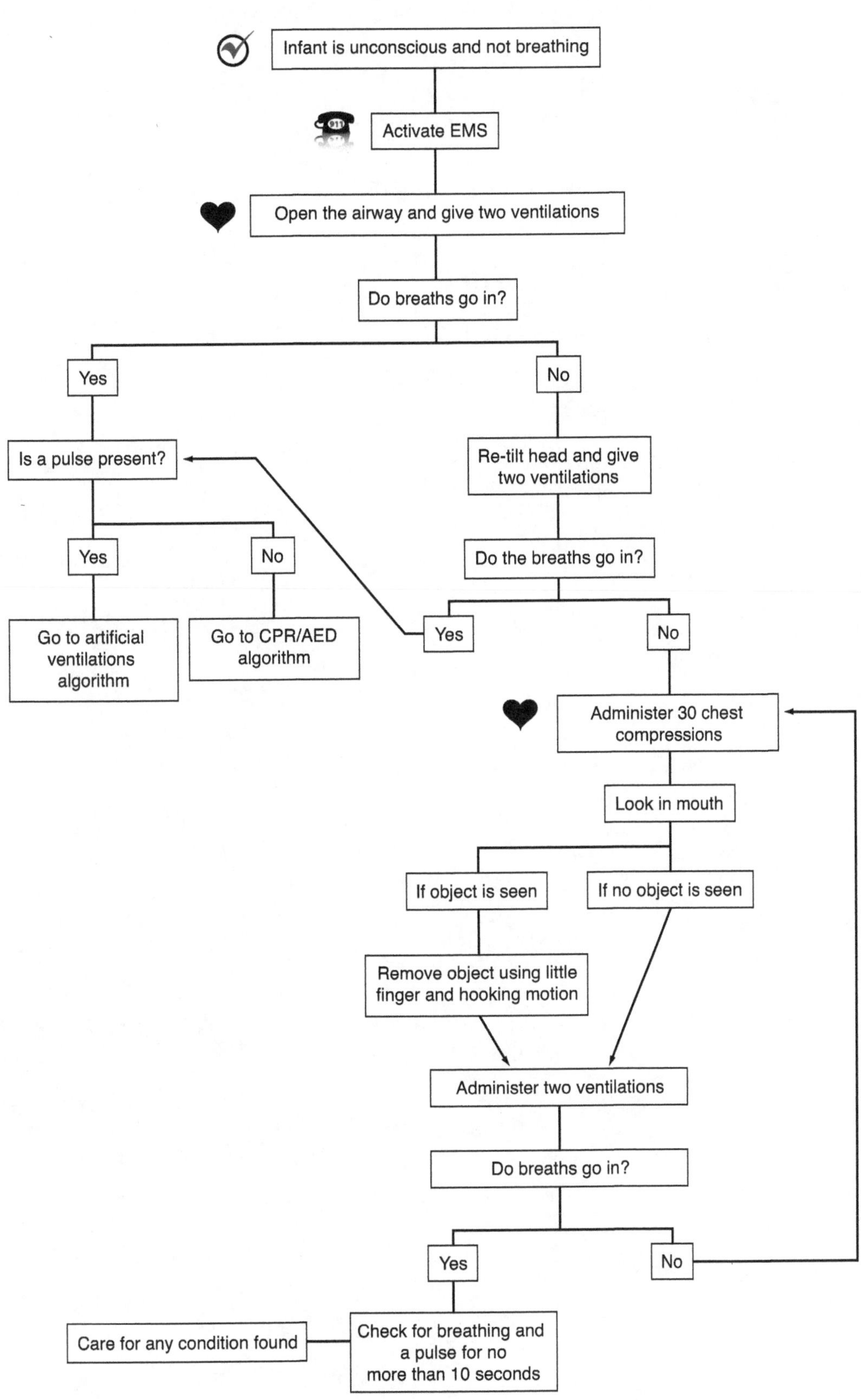
Infant is unconscious and not breathing
Activate EMS
Open the airway and give two ventilations
Do breaths go in?
Yes
No
Is a pulse present?
Re-tilt head and give two ventilations
Yes
No
Do the breaths go in?
Go to artificial ventilations algorithm
Go to CPR/AED algorithm
Yes
No
Administer 30 chest compressions
Look in mouth
If object is seen
If no object is seen
Remove object using little finger and hooking motion
Administer two ventilations
Do breaths go in?
Yes
No
Care for any condition found
Check for breathing and a pulse for no more than 10 seconds

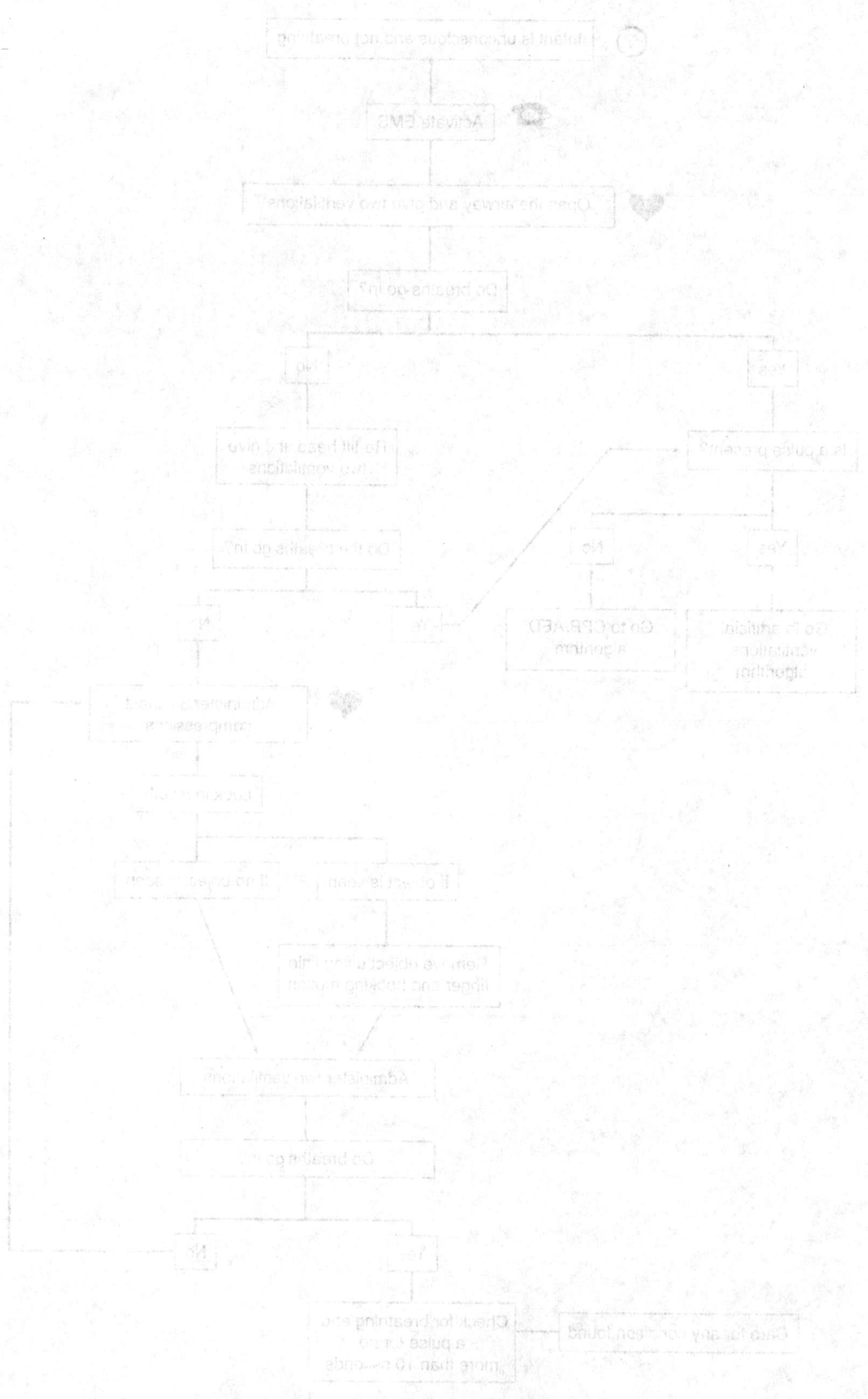

ARTIFICIAL VENTILATIONS—ADULT, CHILD, AND INFANT

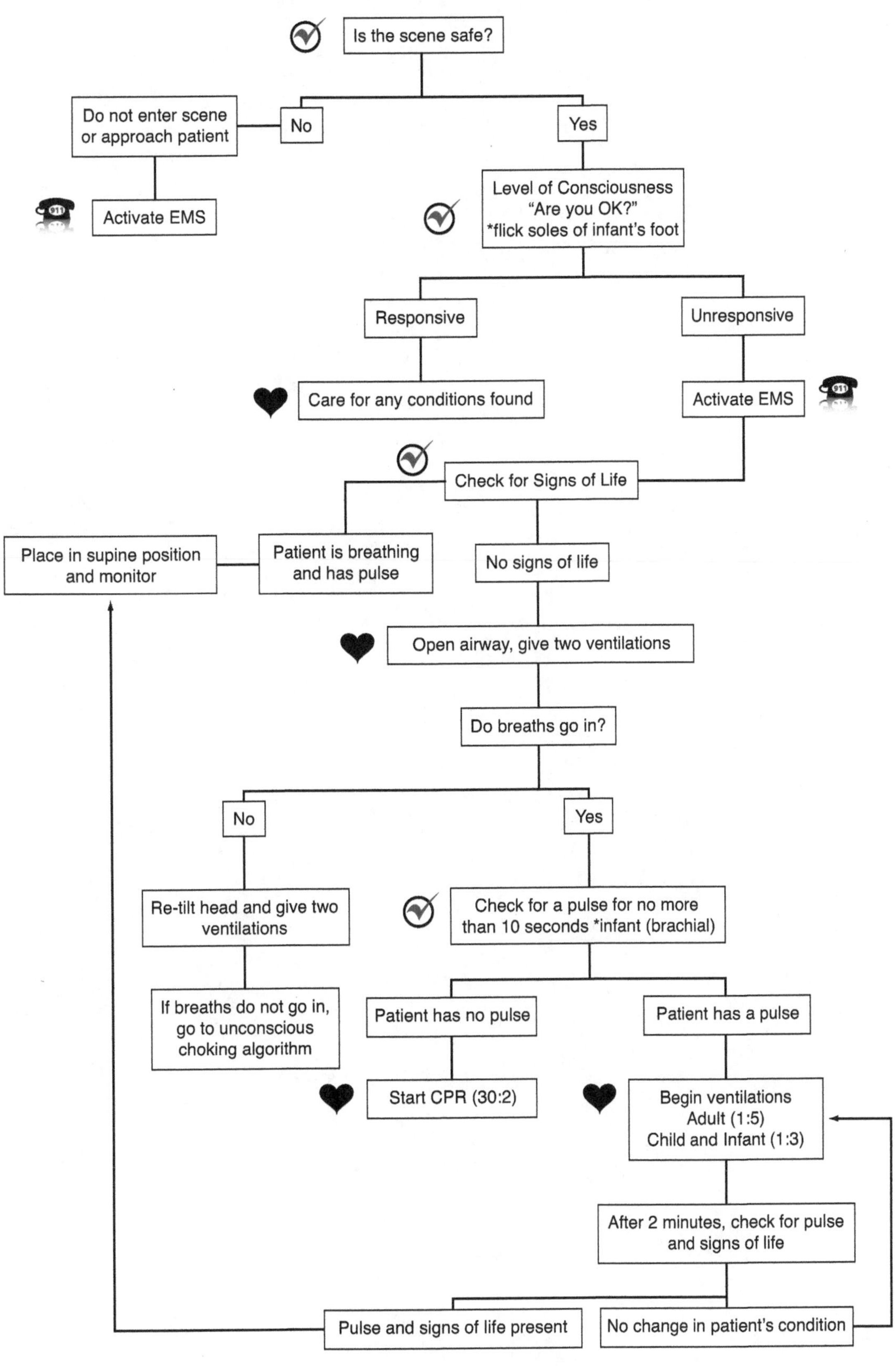

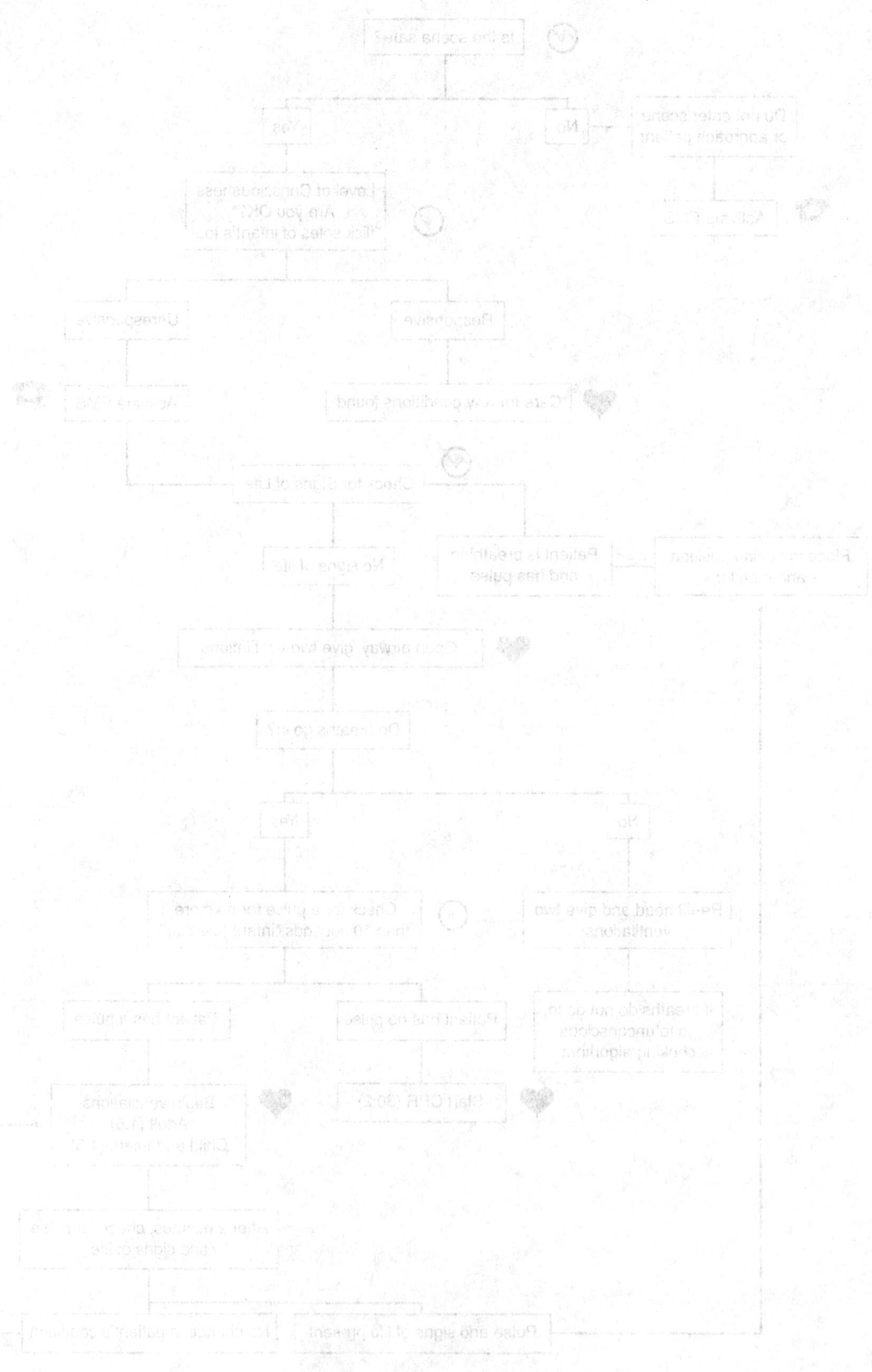

CPR/AED—ADULT

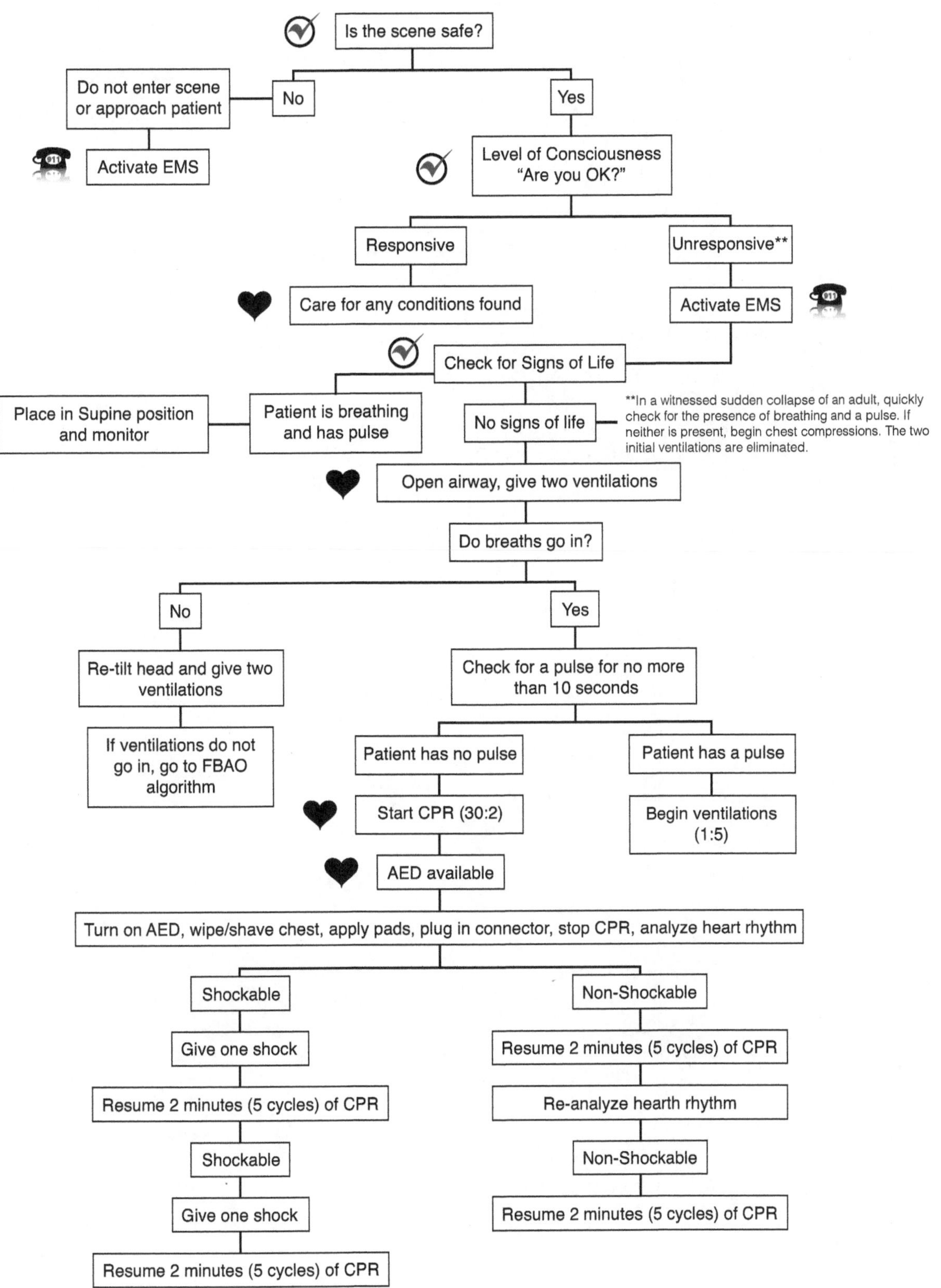

CPR/AED—CHILD AND INFANT

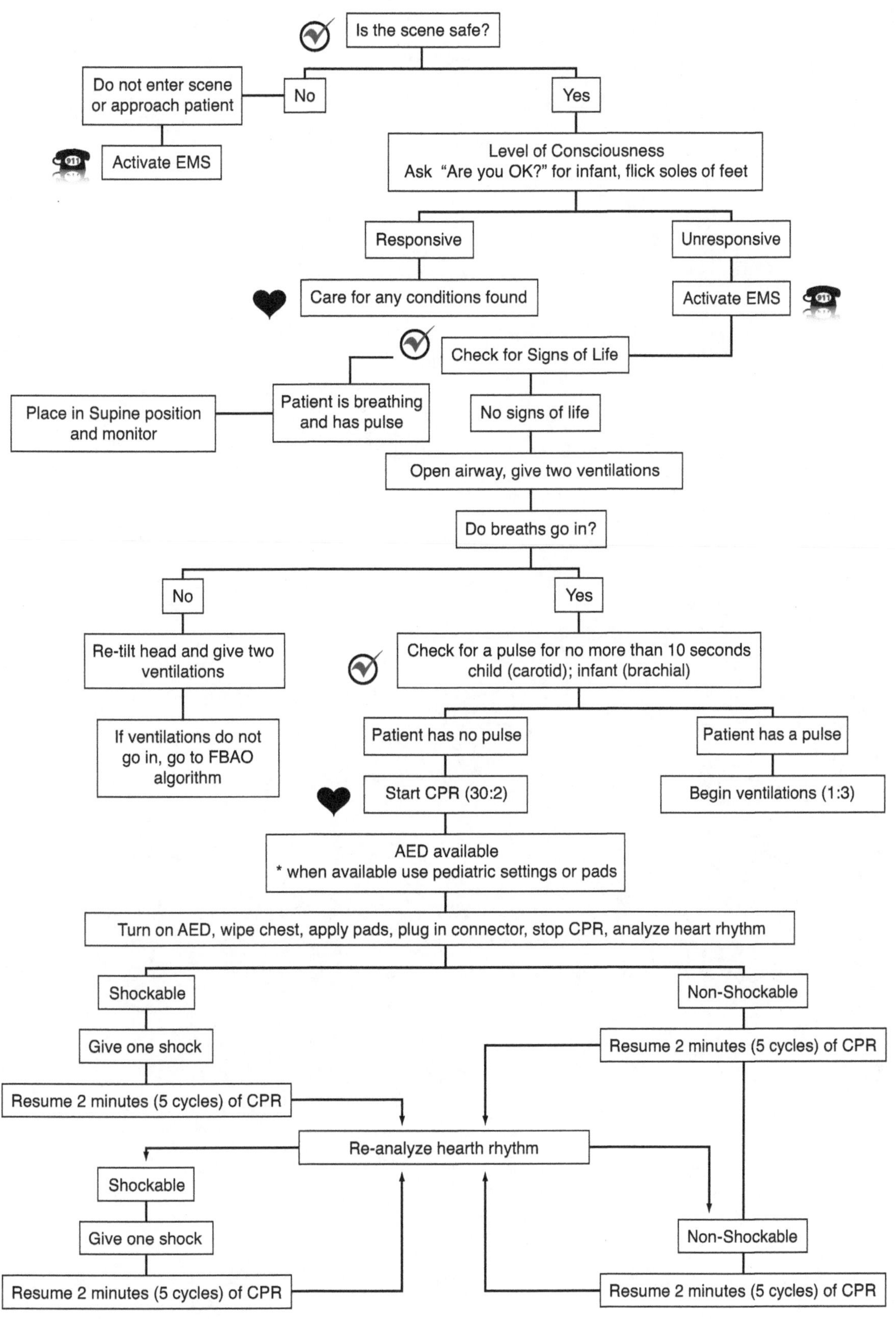